KT-502-635

THE COMPLETE ILLUSTRATED GUIDE TO

REFLEXOLOGY

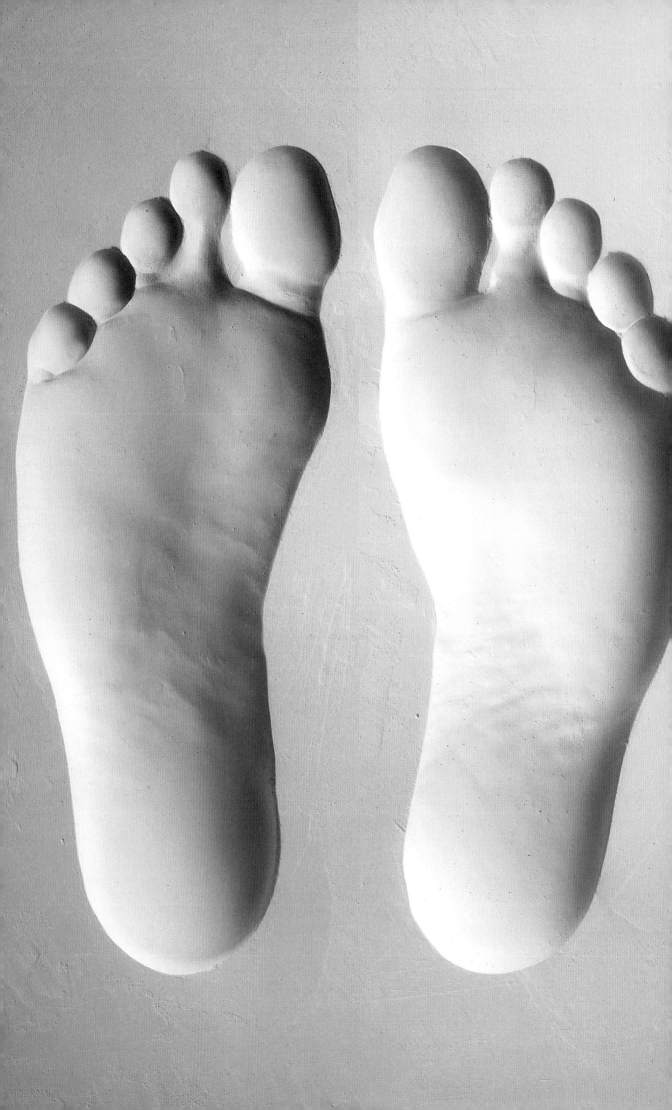

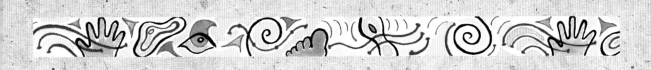

THE COMPLETE
ILLUSTRATED
GUIDE TO

REFLEXOLOGY

Therapeutic Foot Massage
for Health and Well-being

INGE DOUGANS

ELEMENT

Shaftesbury, Dorset • Rockport, Massachusetts • Brisbane, Queensland

© Element Books 1996

Text and techniques © Inge Dougans

First published in Great Britain 1996 by

ELEMENT BOOKS LIMITED

Shaftesbury, Dorset SP7 8BP

Published in USA in 1996 by

ELEMENT BOOKS INC.

PO Box 830, Rockport, MA 01966

Published in Australia in 1996 by

ELEMENT BOOKS LIMITED

for JACARANDA WILEY LIMITED

33 Park Road, Milton, Brisbane 4064

All rights reserved.

No part of this book may be reproduced or utilized
in any form or by any means, electronic or
mechanical, without prior permission in writing
from the Publisher.

NOTE FROM THE PUBLISHER

*Any information given in this book is not intended
to be taken as a replacement for medical advice. Any
person with a condition requiring medical attention
should consult a qualified practitioner or therapist.*

Designed and created for Element Books by

THE BRIDGEWATER BOOK COMPANY

Art Director: **Peter Bridgewater**

Designer: **Andrew Milne**

Mac Artworker: **Amanda Payne**

Managing Editor: **Anne Townley**

Picture research: **Vanessa Fletcher**

Three-dimensional models: **Mark Jamieson**

Studio photography: **Guy Ryecart**

Illustrators: **Paul Allen,
Alan and Gill Bridgewater, Lorraine Harrison,
Andrew Kulman, Andrew Milne**

Printed and bound in the UK
by Butler and Tanner Ltd

British Library Cataloguing in Publication
data available

Library of Congress Cataloging in Publication
data available

ISBN 1 85230 874 5 HARDBACK

ISBN 1 85230 910 5 PAPERBACK

ACKNOWLEDGMENTS

The publishers wish to thank the following for the use of pictures:

Horizon: pp.58 TL (Peter Fyfe), 58M (R. Parker)

Hulton Deutsch Collection: p.58TR

Hutchison Library: p.55 (Sarah Errington)

The Image Bank: pp.11BL (Grant V. Faint), 19R(L. D. Gordon),

Mansell Collection: p.50T

National Medical Slide Bank: pp.101BL, 101BR, 107TL, 113B

The Royal Collection © Her Majesty The Queen: p.48

Science Photo Library: pp.28R (CNRI), 29L (CNRI/G. Hadjo),
30BR (Alfred Pasieka), 31BL (John Sanford), 100T (Francoise
Sauze), 100M (Dr P. Marazzi), 100B (Biophoto Associates), 101T
and 102T (Dr H. C. Robinson), 102M (Dr P. Marazzi), 102B
(James Stevenson), 104L (Biophoto Associates), 104R (Jane
Shemilt), 106T (Dr. Jeremy Burgess), 106M, 106B, 107BL and
108L (Dr P. Marazzi), 108R (Dr H. C. Robinson), 109TL (Dr P.
Marazzi), 109BL, 111L, 112T, 113T and 113M (Dr P. Marazzi)

The Trustee of the Wellcome Trust: pp.49, 54TR

Special thanks go to:

Caroline Dorling and Flint House, Lewes, East Sussex
for help and advice in the preparation of this book

The Kristine Walker School of Reflexology, East Sussex

**Glyn Bridgewater / Lorinda Cronje / Nina Downey
Breeda Duggan / Delores and Isaac Everett
Marianne Hillier-Brook / Simon Holden
Susan and Gina Jamieson / Arthur Larkin
Sarah Mellish / Gwen Musdaw / Clare Packman
Sarah Stanley / Samantha and Eleanor Tuffnell-Smith
Daniel Walker / Jacoba Elizabeth van Der Walt
Tjaart van Der Walt**
for help with photography

The Body Shop and **Cos-tec**

Bright Ideas, Lewes, East Sussex

The Brighton Pine Co, Brighton, East Sussex

Brighton University, East Sussex

Hanningtons Ltd, Brighton, East Sussex

Scholl Consumer Products Ltd, London

Tie Rack, London
for help with properties

Royal Brompton Hospital, London

Douglas Carnall M.R.C.G.P.
for technical and medical advice

Marie van Der Walt
for research for the case studies on pages 114–119

Contents

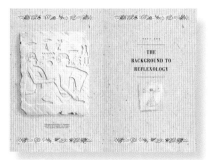

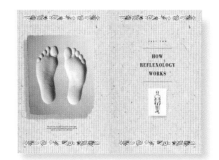

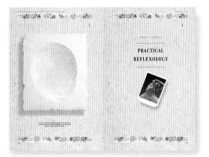

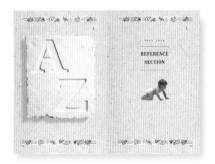

HOW TO USE THIS BOOK

*T*he *Complete Illustrated Guide to Reflexology* is designed as a comprehensive introduction to the art of reflexology giving practical advice about how it can be used as a holistic healing process. The book can be used both as a guide to the benefits that may be expected from a course of reflexology treatment and as an aid to the study of the treatment sequence itself.

Throughout the book the author relates the study of reflexology and the use of massage techniques to the wealth of knowledge contained in Chinese medicine about the circulation of energy in the body through meridians.

The first part of the book, "The Background to Reflexology," explores the place of reflexology in the healing process. The reflexologist can only be one half of a healing partnership – the will to overcome dis-ease has to come from the patient. Sources of stress are explored and methods of counteracting it in our lives are discussed. The role of energy as the basis of life and a factor in healing is examined, and reflexology is placed in the context of zone and meridian therapy.

A detailed study of "How Reflexology Works" is contained in the second part of the book. Here a thorough analysis of reflexology and the meridians is given. Each of the 12 main meridians is examined in depth, and the likely symptoms of congestions along their paths are explained. By combining this knowledge with an understanding of the reflex areas on the foot and how these are related to different organs of the body, also explored in this section, the reflexologist can provide a complete treatment.

The third part of the book contains a detailed step-by-step guide to "Practical Reflexology." The grips and pressure techniques that form the basis of the reflexology treatment are explained through clear color photographs, together with accompanying relaxation techniques. The full-treatment sequence is then shown step-by-step, working from the toes through to the heel of the foot. A summary chart on pages 146–147 provides an at-a-glance guide to the order of treatment and the grips and pressure techniques used to work each set of reflexes.

BELOW

VARIOUS SYMBOLS ARE USED THROUGHOUT THE BOOK FOR EASE OF REFERENCE.

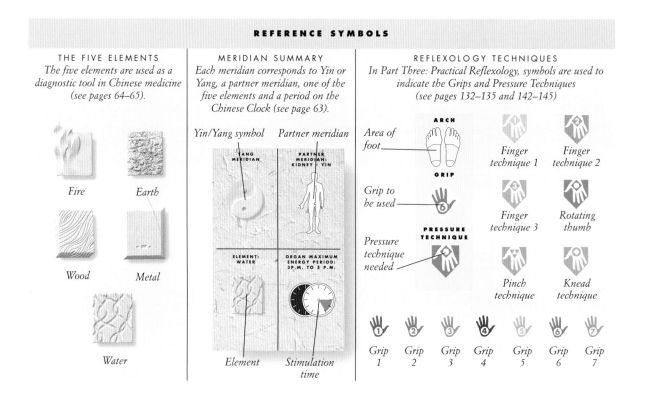

REFERENCE SYMBOLS

THE FIVE ELEMENTS
The five elements are used as a diagnostic tool in Chinese medicine (see pages 64–65).

Fire   Earth

Wood   Metal

Water

MERIDIAN SUMMARY
Each meridian corresponds to Yin or Yang, a partner meridian, one of the five elements and a period on the Chinese Clock (see page 63).

Yin/Yang symbol   Partner meridian

YANG MERIDIAN   PARTNER MERIDIAN: KIDNEY – YIN

ELEMENT: WATER   ORGAN MAXIMUM ENERGY PERIOD: 3 P.M. TO 5 P.M.

Element   Stimulation time

REFLEXOLOGY TECHNIQUES
In Part Three: Practical Reflexology, symbols are used to indicate the Grips and Pressure Techniques (see pages 132–135 and 142–145)

ARCH

Area of foot

GRIP

Grip to be used

PRESSURE TECHNIQUE

Pressure technique needed

Finger technique 1   Finger technique 2

Finger technique 3   Rotating thumb

Pinch technique   Knead technique

Grip 1   Grip 2   Grip 3   Grip 4   Grip 5   Grip 6   Grip 7

Visual reference guide to each meridian's cycle, partner meridian, element, and energy time.

Text examining the path of each meridian through the body.

Case studies showing how reflexology can combat disorders along the meridians.

Main text explaining the patient's role in the healing process.

Clear graphics and original photography outlining the holistic path to health.

Quick graphic reference guide to the grips and techniques used.

Clear step-by-step photography showing how to work each reflex of the foot.

Life-size photographic details for greater clarity.

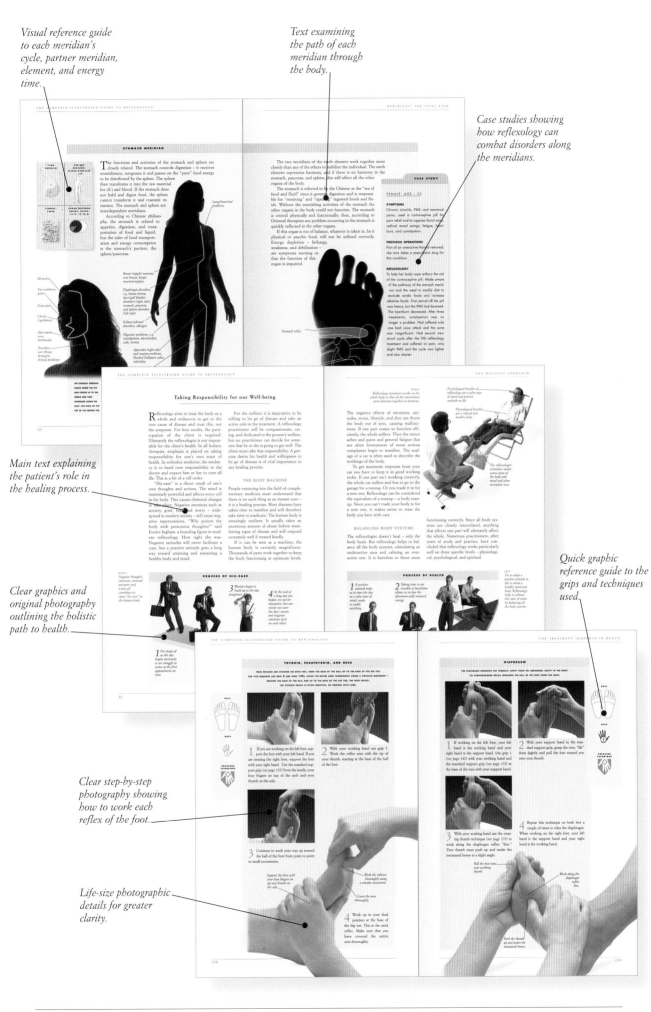

INTRODUCTION

Reflexology is a gentle art, a fascinating science, and an extremely effective form of therapeutic foot massage that has carved an impressive niche in the field of alternative medicine. It is a science because it is based on physiological and neurological study; it is an art because much depends on how skillfully the practitioner applies his or her knowledge, and the dynamics that occur between practitioner and recipient.[1]

Reflexology is a holistic healing technique – the term "holistic" derived from the Greek word holos, which means "whole" – and as such aims to treat the individual as an entity, incorporating body, mind, and spirit. Reflexologists do not isolate a disease and treat it symptomatically, nor do they work specifically on a problem organ or system, but on the whole person with the object of inducing a state of balance and of harmony.

The art of reflex foot massage must not be confused with basic foot massage or body massage in general. It is a specific pressure technique that works on precise reflex points on the feet, based on the premise that reflex areas on the feet correspond with all body parts. Because the feet represent a microcosm of the body, all organs, glands, and other body parts are laid out in a similar arrangement on the feet.

ABOVE
As a holistic healing technique, reflexology treats all the individual pieces of a person as a whole – mind, body, and spirit.

1 – CHRISTINE ISSEL "REFLEXOLOGY: ART, SCIENCE AND HISTORY" P122

RIGHT
The feet provide an easily accessible microcosm of the entire body.

The phenomenon of micro-cosmic representation of body parts in different areas of the body is also evident in the iris of the eye, the ear, and the hands. The corresponding areas on the feet are, however, easier to locate because they cover a larger area and are more specific, rendering them easier to work on. Firm pressure is applied to the relevant reflex area using both specific thumb and finger techniques.

This causes physiological changes to take place in the body since the body's own healing potential is stimulated. Thus, the feet can play a major role in attaining and maintaining better health.

The simplicity of reflexology treatment belies its efficacy. No high-tech, complicated equipment is necessary. The technique is so simple it does not require years of training to master. A good practitioner needs a sensitive but sturdy pair of hands, a genuine desire to ease the client's pain and suffering, compassion, intuition, and an understanding of human nature. The relationship between the recipient and practitioner is an important aspect of the healing process. The practitioner acts as mediator to activate the client's healing potential.

Who Can Benefit from Reflexology?

Reflexology does not discriminate. There are no boundaries or limitations. People of any age or sex – the elderly, women, men, teenagers, children, and babies – can derive positive benefits from reflexology. Reflexology can do no harm, although please remember that caution should be taken with thrombosis (it could move the blood clot) and with diabetes, especially if insulin is being given (if the treat-ment activates the pancreas the insulin level has to be reduced). Other restrictions are those determined by the receiver's pain threshold and his or her reactions to massage. Elderly people with no specific complaint will benefit from a couple of courses of treatment a year to keep bodily functions toned. Results are also good with children and babies because they are more relaxed and supple and because their bodies are highly receptive to therapeutic stimuli.

Reflexology has proved itself to be effective, but because no two people are the same, what may be of great benefit for one person may not have the same results for another. Because reflexology treatment reaches the receiver on several levels – physical, mental, and spiritual – it can only be of benefit.

LEFT
The elderly will find that stiff joints and circulatory problems, in particular, benefit from reflexology treatment.

BELOW
Babies are the most receptive patients because they are naturally relaxed.

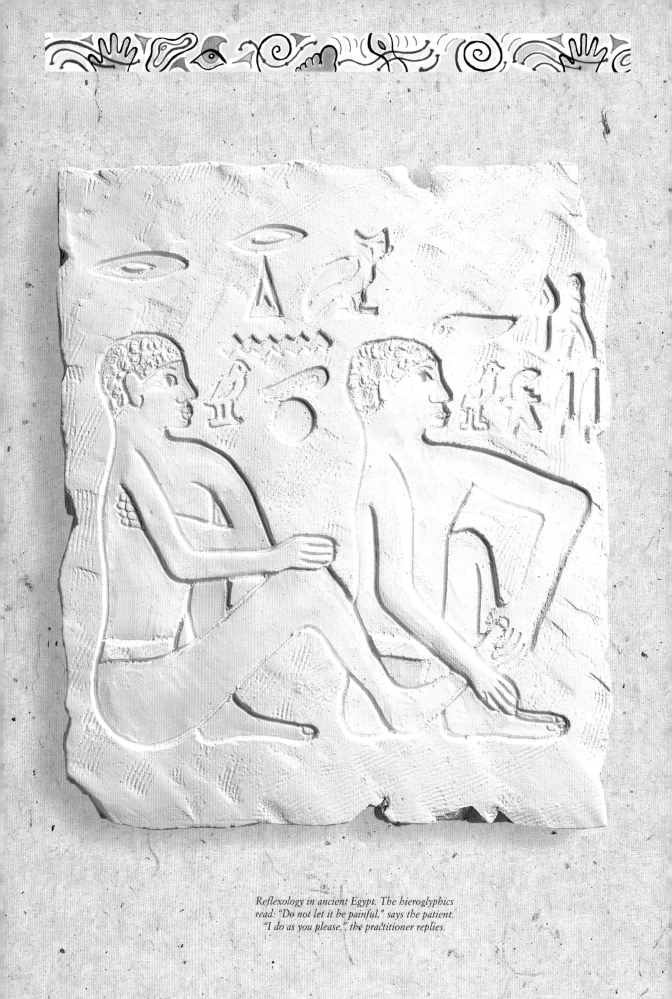

Reflexology in ancient Egypt. The hieroglyphics read: "Do not let it be painful," says the patient. "I do as you please," the practitioner replies.

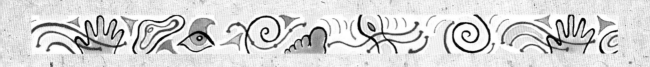

PART ONE

THE BACKGROUND TO REFLEXOLOGY

1. THE HOLISTIC APPROACH

RIGHT
Alternative medicine is based on traditional folk medicine, which used natural herbs and other plants ground into pastes and powders as remedies.

Until relatively recently practitioners of reflexology adopted an approach that was purely physical. Reflexology was seen as an effective way of dealing with physical ailments in the body, but little thought was given to emotional aspects. Now, however, a more "holistic" view is taken, incorporating mind and soul in addition to body – the physical state is widely acknowledged also to reflect the well-being of the emotional mind.

Fire (Eastern)

Earth (Western) *Air (Western)* *Wood (Eastern)* *Metal (Eastern)*

Reflexology – a Branch of Alternative Medicine

Reflexology falls into the realm of alternative medicine. In the modern context this term refers to any form of medicine that does not fall into the mainstream of the orthodox Western approach. This is in fact a misrepresentation. Orthodox medicine is the one that should be referred to as the "alternative" because of its relative infancy in the history of medicinal practices.

Many practices considered "alternative" hail from antiquity and are based on traditional folk medicine that existed in all cultures. Every culture and country had its traditional medical system. In those times medicine was a blend of art and science with a generous sprinkling of magic, myth, and superstition. As "modern" medicine evolved, science took precedence and medicine became mechanical, looking at life as a purely chemical phenomenon. The human body came to be regarded as a machine made up of a complex collection of parts. Natural medical practices were pushed into the background and suppressed.

Several decades down the line, the tables are turning. Disillusionment with modern medicine has resulted in a resurgence of enthusiasm and demand for

Earth (Eastern) *Water (Western)* *Fire (Western)* *Water (Eastern)*

ABOVE
Practitioners of traditional medicine in the East believe that the human body and mind depend on a balance of the five elements for their well-being. In the West, medieval healing looked to the four elements of Earth, Water, Air, and Fire.

safer, more natural forms of therapy. Both orthodox and alternative practices have their place in health care and should ideally work together, since no one therapy can claim to be able to deal with every disease. And neither could claim to be total health care systems. No one can deny the benefits that modern technology can bring, but in the race for better and more expensive treatment a vital aspect of healing – the human element – has often been forced into the background.

The human body is far more than a collection of working parts. It is a highly sophisticated organism imbued with the vital dimensions of body, mind, and spirit. Modern doctors are not always trained to recognize problems beyond the physical. Most therapies, reflexology among them, recognize that physical imbalance seldom occurs in isolation. Imbalance in mental and spiritual spheres cannot be separated from the physical, so intricately are these interwoven. Orthodox medicine sometimes seems not to recognize this interdependence and people become disillusioned as they see it failing in chronic conditions and witness the destructive and disturbing side-effects that some drugs and surgery can have.

MODERN DRUGS

Most modern drugs are manufactured from inorganic chemicals developed in laboratories. We are organic beings with a physiology designed to assimilate organic substances, not manufactured chemicals. Constant ingestion of drugs can eventually only result in negative conditions as toxic residues accumulate. Almost every drug developed has some destructive side-effect on another function of the body. Drugs suppress disease, relieve symptoms, and ease pain but they do not deal with the underlying cause of the "dis-ease" and eradicate that.

Overexposure to drugs has produced a new kind of disease – iatrogenic disease –

illness that is the result of medical or surgical treatment. Exact figures for iatrogenic disease are difficult to assess. Many people do eventually require hospital treatment for this affliction, but there are thousands of victims who battle on through daily life feeling "not quite right," unaware of the root cause of their malaise.

WORKING TOGETHER

There can be no doubt that modern medicine has contributed greatly to the improvement of health care. For example, prior to the advent of penicillin, disease epidemics were devastating. Surgery is another wonder of modern medicine, a miracle of modern technology that provides impressive and life-saving treatment for numerous conditions. But this is not the only answer. As the object of both orthodox and alternative medicine is to cure disease and be of assistance to the human race, the most positive prognosis would be that both recognize their place in health care and work together for the benefit of all.

The best alternative therapies combined with the finest in technological medicine would be a great breakthrough in health care. To quote a World Health Organization report: "for too long traditional systems of medicine and 'modern' medicine have gone their separate ways in mutual antipathy. Yet are not their goals identical – to improve the health of mankind and thereby the quality of life? Only the blinkered mind would assume that each has nothing to do with the other."[1] Reflexology has a major part to play in this wider vision of health care.

BELOW
Modern medicine with its increasingly sophisticated instrumentation, techniques, and drugs has enabled many medical conditions to be cured and improved, but it can also have harmful side-effects.

1 – ANDREW STANWAY, M.B., M.R.C.P. "ALTERNATIVE MEDICINE" P.36

Taking Responsibility for our Well-being

Reflexology aims to treat the body as a whole and endeavors to get to the root cause of disease and treat this, not the symptom. For best results, the participation of the client is required. Ultimately the reflexologist is not responsible for the client's health. In all holistic therapies, emphasis is placed on taking responsibility for one's own state of health. In orthodox medicine, the tendency is to hand over responsibility to the doctor and expect him or her to cure all ills. This is a bit of a tall order.

"Dis-ease" is a direct result of one's own thoughts and actions. The mind is immensely powerful and affects every cell in the body. This causes chemical changes to take place. Negative emotions such as anxiety, grief, fear, and worry – widespread in modern society – will cause negative repercussions. "Why poison the body with poisonous thoughts?" said Eunice Ingham, a founding figure in modern reflexology. How right she was. Negative attitudes will never facilitate a cure, but a positive attitude goes a long way toward attaining and sustaining a healthy body and mind.

For the sufferer it is imperative to be willing to let go of disease and take an active role in the treatment. A reflexology practitioner will be compassionate, caring, and dedicated to the person's welfare, but no practitioner can decide for someone that he or she is going to get well. The client must take that responsibility. A genuine desire for health and willingness to let go of disease is of vital importance to any healing process.

THE BODY MACHINE

People venturing into the field of complementary medicine must understand that there is no such thing as an instant cure – it is a healing process. Most diseases have taken time to manifest and will therefore take time to eradicate. The human body is amazingly resilient. It usually takes an enormous amount of abuse before manifesting signs of disease and will respond extremely well if treated kindly.

If it can be seen as a machine, the human body is certainly magnificent. Thousands of parts work together to keep the body functioning at optimum levels.

RIGHT
Negative thoughts, emotions, external pressures and worry all contribute to cause "dis-ease" in the human body.

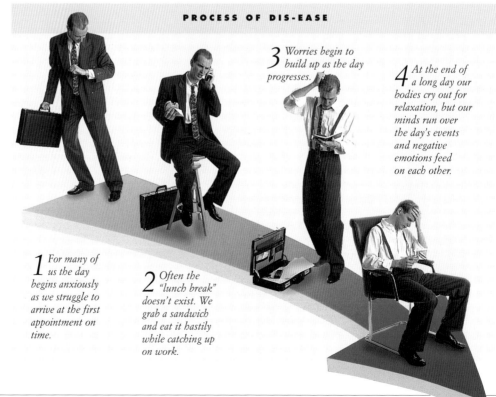

PROCESS OF DIS-EASE

3 Worries begin to build up as the day progresses.

4 At the end of a long day our bodies cry out for relaxation, but our minds run over the day's events and negative emotions feed on each other.

1 For many of us the day begins anxiously as we struggle to arrive at the first appointment on time.

2 Often the "lunch break" doesn't exist. We grab a sandwich and eat it hastily while catching up on work.

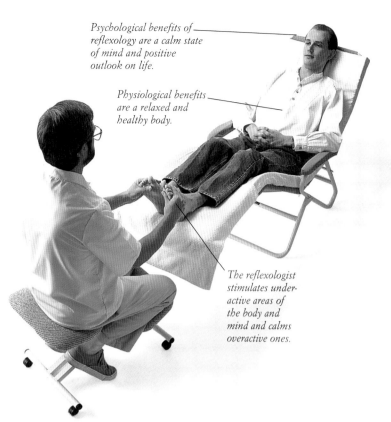

RIGHT
Reflexology treatment works on the whole body so that all the interrelated parts function together in harmony.

Psychological benefits of reflexology are a calm state of mind and positive outlook on life.

Physiological benefits are a relaxed and healthy body.

The reflexologist stimulates under-active areas of the body and mind and calms overactive ones.

The negative effects of emotions, attitudes, stress, lifestyle, and diet can throw the body out of sync, causing malfunctions. If one part ceases to function efficiently, the whole suffers. Then the minor aches and pains and general fatigue that are often forerunners of more serious complaints begin to manifest. The analogy of a car is often used to describe the workings of the body.

To get maximum response from your car you have to keep it in good working order. If one part isn't working correctly, the whole car suffers and has to go to the garage for a tuneup. Or you trade it in for a new one. Reflexology can be considered the equivalent of a tuneup – a body tuneup. Since you can't trade your body in for a new one, it makes sense to treat the body you have with care.

BALANCING BODY SYSTEMS

The reflexologist doesn't heal – only the body heals. But reflexology helps to balance all the body systems, stimulating an underactive area and calming an overactive one. It is harmless to those areas functioning correctly. Since all body systems are closely interrelated, anything that affects one part will ultimately affect the whole. Numerous practitioners, after years of study and practice, have concluded that reflexology works particularly well on three specific levels – physiological, psychological, and spiritual.

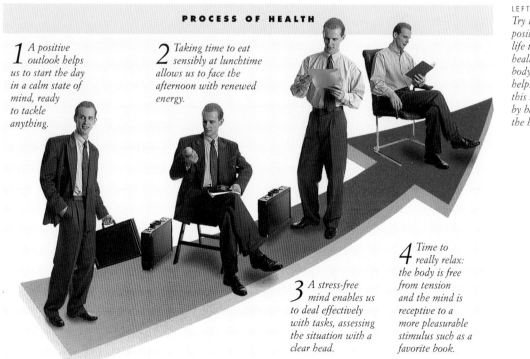

PROCESS OF HEALTH

1 A positive outlook helps us to start the day in a calm state of mind, ready to tackle anything.

2 Taking time to eat sensibly at lunchtime allows us to face the afternoon with renewed energy.

3 A stress-free mind enables us to deal effectively with tasks, assessing the situation with a clear head.

4 Time to really relax: the body is free from tension and the mind is receptive to a more pleasurable stimulus such as a favorite book.

LEFT
Try to adopt a positive attitude to life to attain a healthy mind and body. Reflexology helps to achieve this state of mind by balancing all the body systems.

Maintaining a Positive and Balanced Lifestyle

RIGHT
Human body cells are replaced regularly. Every year 98 percent of our bodies is completely renewed.

People in the West often take their health for granted and abuse it in many different ways. For thousands of years it was accepted that illness resulted from a disturbance in our internal environment. Then came the orthodox scientific approach dominated by the germ theory. This theory evolved from the findings of French chemist and biologist Louis Pasteur, the founder of bacteriology. It has been the focus of modern forms of medicine ever since.

Microorganisms may be involved in many ailments but their presence does not automatically guarantee disease. We are surrounded by numerous disease-bearing organisms, but only a fraction of the people exposed to these succumb to any form of infection. For example, if three people breathe the same germs at the same time, one may develop pneumonia, another a cold, and the third may never be aware that the germs were there.

STATE OF MIND

Disease is generated by a combination of circumstances both inside and outside the body. The main object of holistic healing is to help correct the life condition that predisposes a person to disease. A number of factors can initiate disease, the most important of which is state of mind.

The mind is immensely powerful and the relationship between mind and body should never be underestimated. Because all life is based on energy, health is considered to be the harmonious interplay of energies within the body. Negative thoughts and emotions restrict the free flow of these energies, causing congestions that ultimately manifest as disease if not corrected. It is now widely accepted that a positive attitude is a major step toward creating a healthy body. This general theory is most eloquently expressed by Dr. Randolph Stone who said: "As you think, so you are."

All thoughts and emotions reverberate throughout every cell in the body and manifest physiologically. For example, the

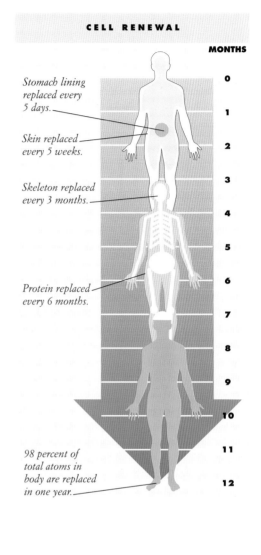

CELL RENEWAL

MONTHS

Stomach lining replaced every 5 days.

Skin replaced every 5 weeks.

Skeleton replaced every 3 months.

Protein replaced every 6 months.

0
1
2
3
4
5
6
7
8
9
10
11
12

98 percent of total atoms in body are replaced in one year.

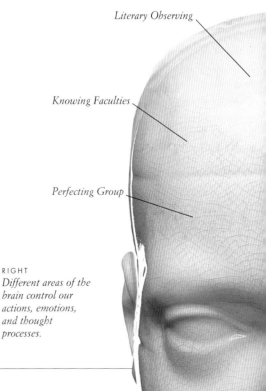

Literary Observing

Knowing Faculties

Perfecting Group

RIGHT
Different areas of the brain control our actions, emotions, and thought processes.

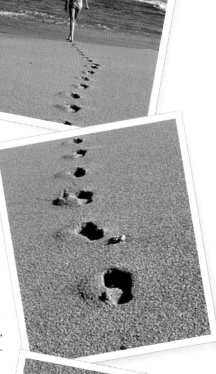

angry and disturbed person develops an acid system, a preponderance of the positively charged H[+] ion.[2] Emotions also alter endocrine balance, impair blood supply and blood pressure, impede digestion, change body temperature, and produce a sustained state of emotional stress, causing physiological changes that lead to disease.[3] Illness is a natural expression of what is happening inside the body. It is pointless to treat this with superficial drugs designed to suppress the problem because the seat of the disease may be in a different part of the body from the one in which it manifests.

CREATING A "NEW" BODY

The human body is composed of about 1 trillion cells all working toward a common end – the maintenance of a healthy individual.[4] These body cells are constantly changing. The materials of our bodies and brains are renewed regularly. All the protein in the body is replaced every six months and in some organs, such as the liver, the protein is renewed more frequently.[5] We acquire a new stomach lining every five days (the innermost layer of stomach cells is exchanged in a matter of

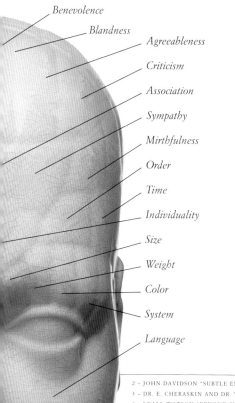

Benevolence
Blandness
Agreeableness
Criticism
Association
Sympathy
Mirthfulness
Order
Time
Individuality
Size
Weight
Color
System
Language

minutes as food is digested). Skin is new every five weeks. The skeleton is entirely new every three months. Every year 98 percent of the total number of atoms in the body are replaced.[6] And at the end of each seven-year period, every cell in the body has been replaced.

As old cells die and disappear, instead of replacing them with cells programmed with the same negative thoughts and fed on inadequate nutrition, one should learn to reprogram them with positive, nutritious information to create a "new" being. This is not impossible. It just requires sustained dedicated effort and the genuine desire for health.

Every person has the potential for perfect health. It may require effort and dedication, but the rewards are often tremendous. Dr. Stone sums up admirably the state of true "health" that reflexology and all truly holistic therapies have as their goal: "Health is not merely of the body. It is the natural expression of the body, mind and soul when they are in rhythm with the One Life. True health is the harmony of life within us, consisting of peace of mind, happiness and well-being. It is not merely a question of physical fitness, but is rather the result of the soul finding free expression through the mind and body of that individual. Such a person radiates peace and happiness and everyone in his presence automatically feels happy and contented."[7]

ABOVE
Footprints give a good indication of the state of body, and mind: these are firm and well-balanced indicating a healthy body, and enthusiasm and energy for life.

2 – JOHN DAVIDSON "SUBTLE ENERGY" P126
3 – DR. E. CHERASKIN AND DR. W.M. RINGSDORF, JR. WITH ARLINE BRECHER "PSYCHODIETETICS" P17
4 – LYALL WATSON "BEYOND SUPERNATURE" P117   5 – HAROLD SAXTON BURR "BLUEPRINT FOR IMMORTALITY" P12
6 – DEEPAK CHOPRA, M.D., "PERFECT HEALTH" P12   7 – FRANKLYN SILLS "THE POLARITY PROCESS" P91

2. COUNTERACTING STRESS

*I*n our modern rushed and demanding lifestyle we are susceptible to a continual buildup of tension, anxiety, and fear. However, stress is manufactured within our bodies, not absorbed from external forces.

Reflexology expels the suppressed emotions of stress, relaxing both our bodies and our attitudes to life.

BELOW
A relaxed body reflected in the face: muscles relax, hard lines disappear, and the expression is happy and contented.

Reflexology and Relaxation

One of the most important benefits of reflexology is its efficacy in reducing stress.

Approximately 70 percent of disorders can be related to stress and nerve tension. Because reflexology encourages the body to relax, other functions are also affected. Every part of the body receives its nerve supply direct from the spine. Abnormal tension leads to tightening of the muscles of the spine; thus nerves are affected, resulting in pain. When tension is relaxed, the muscles cease to contract. Blood vessels too are relaxed, reducing vascular constriction and allowing circulation to flow freely, thereby conducting the necessary oxygen and nutrients to all the body tissues and organs. This in turn helps cleanse the body of toxins and impurities.

Stress is difficult to avoid. It is an integral part of modern life. The days when the stress syndrome was associated only with high-powered business executives are long gone. Today young children,

women, men, and the elderly are all subject to varying degrees of stress. Survival in our fast-paced century is stressful. The speed of change and modern technology contribute to major malfunctions in body and psyche. The barrage of "stressors" is unrelenting – traffic, television, noise, job pressure, family problems, wars, famines, disease, environmental problems, electronic smog, financial problems, global problems, pollution – the list is endless.

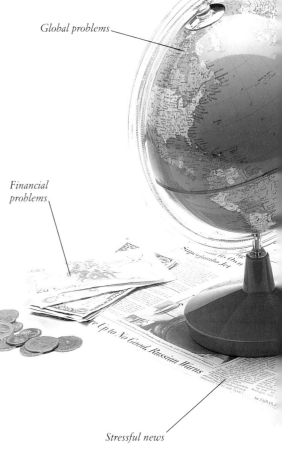

Global problems

Financial problems

Stressful news

STRESS-RELATED DISEASE

Few people escape the consequences of stress. The increasing number of people with heart disease and high blood pressure is evidence of the more obvious stress-related diseases. Other symptoms, though more nebulous, can also be deadly. Long-term symptoms of constant exposure to stress are fatigue, anxiety, and depression. The nervous system becomes drained and depleted, and the immune system eroded, making one more susceptible to immunodeficiency diseases.

Not all stress is negative. It can be immensely stimulating. The human body is equipped to cope with short-term invigorating stress. But long-term constant exposure to stress is devastating.

Stress affects different people in different ways and to varying degrees. One person may exhibit cardiovascular problems, another gastrointestinal upset, anorexia, palpitations, sweating, or headaches – to mention but a few of the myriad body reactions. The cardiovascular and digestive systems are targets for the ill effects of stress – high blood pressure, ulcers, and indigestion being obvious results. Stress can also be linked to infectious diseases. When the body is busy dealing with the effects of residual stress, it cannot organize an effective defense against invading organisms.[1]

LEARNING TO RELAX

Reflexology helps to alleviate the effects of stress by inducing deep relaxation, thereby allowing the nervous system to function normally and free the body to seek its own homeostasis. Reflexology is a powerful antidote to stress. A relaxed body can heal itself, and reflexology is a guaranteed method of relaxing the body and balancing the biological systems. Initial response to reflexology massage varies. Ultimately there will be a surge of vitality and well-being. The overall sensation will then extend to take over the mind and the subconscious. Reflexology means taking that positive step to release the mind from its shackles, enabling the recipient to become him– or herself, thinking positively in order to exclude ill-health.

For hypertension and anxiety, choose reflexology – it is a safe way to induce relaxation and does not have any unpleasant side-effects.

BELOW
Stress shows on the face as muscles tense causing hard lines, and the expression is fixed in a frown.

Family pressures

Pollution

ABOVE
Our modern world is a minefield of stress-inducing factors that can affect everyone from the very young to the very old.

The Mechanisms of Stress

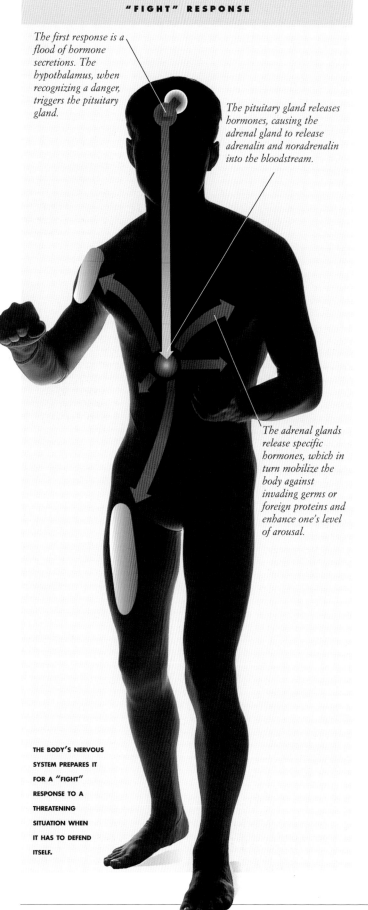

"FIGHT" RESPONSE

The first response is a flood of hormone secretions. The hypothalamus, when recognizing a danger, triggers the pituitary gland.

The pituitary gland releases hormones, causing the adrenal gland to release adrenalin and noradrenalin into the bloodstream.

The adrenal glands release specific hormones, which in turn mobilize the body against invading germs or foreign proteins and enhance one's level of arousal.

THE BODY'S NERVOUS SYSTEM PREPARES IT FOR A "FIGHT" RESPONSE TO A THREATENING SITUATION WHEN IT HAS TO DEFEND ITSELF.

The stress reaction is a primitive response to a threatening or dangerous situation, and has been of essential importance in ensuring the continued survival of the human species. We are the product of thousands of years of evolution. Our survival has depended on quick physical responses to dangers, and the stress reaction is commonly referred to as the "fight-or-flight" reaction.

In primitive times, this burst of energy was utilized in physical activity such as a life-or-death struggle or a quick dash to safety. Today these responses would be considered largely unacceptable in many cultures. To attack the boss or a sales clerk for causing you stress would invariably result in legal repercussions, while fleeing from a tense meeting would be perceived as a mental aberration.

THEORIES OF STRESS RESPONSE

Until recently it was believed that all stress was a result of external forces exerting pressure on an individual. This does not explain why, when confronted by similar situations, one person will react calmly while another may be completely devastated. More recent theories emphasize that the stress response depends on the interaction between a person and his or her environment. The intensity of the stress experience is determined by how a person feels he or she can cope with an identified threat.

The hormonal and chemical defense mechanisms that evolved over the centuries as a means of protection have been retained, but today they have little outlet. The inability to express any physical response to a stressful situation means that our natural instincts are suppressed, which can cause dire harm.

What exactly are the physiological effects of stress? When confronted by a situation we perceive as threatening, our thoughts regarding ourselves and the situation trigger two branches of the central nervous system – the sympathetic and parasympathetic systems.

The sympathetic nervous system initiates involuntary responses designed to activate all the major systems of the body. The first response is a flood of hormone secretions. The hypothalamus, when recognizing a danger, triggers the pituitary gland. This gland releases hormones that cause the adrenal gland to intensify the output of adrenalin and noradrenalin into the bloodstream. These two hormones mimic the actions of nervous stimulation in a number of organs in the body. Although any number of factors can trigger the adrenocortical stress reaction, the response itself is always the same. It involves the release from the adrenal glands of specific hormones, mainly the corticosteroids, which in turn mobilize the body against invading germs or foreign proteins and enhance one's level of arousal. The stress response always activates the immune system.

PHYSIOLOGICAL RESPONSE

The stress chemicals induce physiological changes designed to improve performance. Blood supply to the brain is increased, initially improving judgment and decision making. The heart speeds up and fuel is released into the bloodstream from glucose, fats, or stored blood sugar to provide additional energy. More blood is sent to the muscles to allow for instant action. Breathing rate and function improve as air passages relax. A sense of stimulation is produced and blood pressure rises. Because digestion and excretion are not considered high priorities in a "dangerous" situation, adrenalin causes vascular constriction, which reduces the flow of blood to the stomach and intestine. Blood vessels dilate in some areas and constrict in others; for example, blood is drained from the skin to make it available for use in other areas of the body such as the muscles.

When the body prepares for "fight-or-flight," it is ready for a short burst of heightened activity. In modern society numerous factors can trigger this

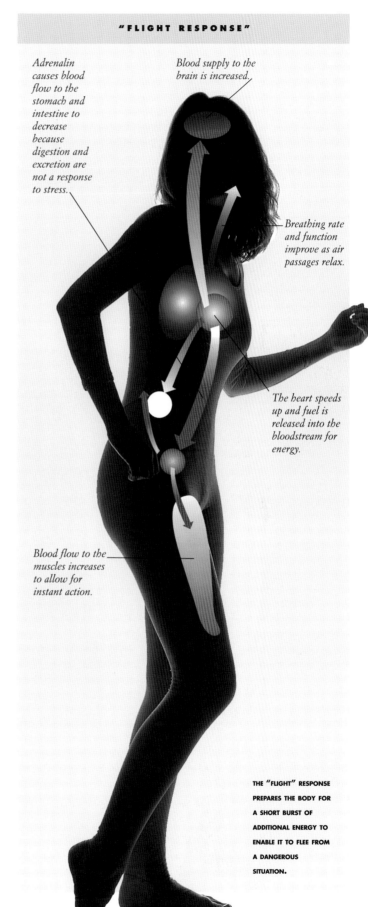

"FLIGHT RESPONSE"

Adrenalin causes blood flow to the stomach and intestine to decrease because digestion and excretion are not a response to stress.

Blood supply to the brain is increased.

Breathing rate and function improve as air passages relax.

The heart speeds up and fuel is released into the bloodstream for energy.

Blood flow to the muscles increases to allow for instant action.

THE "FLIGHT" RESPONSE PREPARES THE BODY FOR A SHORT BURST OF ADDITIONAL ENERGY TO ENABLE IT TO FLEE FROM A DANGEROUS SITUATION.

response, but few can be dealt with by a short burst of activity. Often stress situations are continuous so stress responses are semipermanently on red alert, but physical release is usually unacceptable, so this is all suppressed – a situation that cannot be maintained for too long. The stress buildup eventually explodes internally, knocks the body systems out of balance and causes extreme physical and mental exhaustion.

RESPONSE TO CONTINUAL STRESS

The role of the parasympathetic nervous system is to relax the body after a stressful encounter. However, if a person is subject to continuous stress, it becomes more difficult to activate the parasympathetic reaction. If the stress situation continues unabated, the body itself weakens and becomes more susceptible to a variety of diseases.

Long-term adrenal stimulation with no discharges of energy will deplete essential minerals and vitamins from the system, for example Vitamins B and C, which are vital for the functioning of the immune system.[2] This will result in lowered resistance and increased susceptibility to disease directly related to the immune system such as ME.

Long-term adrenal accumulation can also affect blood pressure and cause a buildup of fatty substances on blood vessel walls, as well as damaging the functioning of the digestive system.

When an organism faces a continual or repeated stress, the response system enters the chronic phase, during which the body's normal resistance declines below normal and becomes exhausted. Several diseases result directly from this chronic stage, but the most important effect is a decrease in the body's ability to fight infection and also to fight cancer.[3]

Everyone is confronted daily with potentially stressful situations. One's vulnerability to stress can be influenced by life events that cause undue emotional strain. Emotional distress is one resistance–lowering factor. Another important factor, according to some health professionals, is the impact of major life changes such as birth, death, marriage, and also increasingly divorce.

The extent to which events lead to ill health, however, will depend to a large degree on a person's capacity to cope with stress. The way an individual perceives a situation will dramatically affect the stress response experienced. It is not so much the *actual* ability to cope with a situation that matters as the individual's *perception* of his or her ability to cope.

It is believed that up to 70 percent of modern diseases have a background that is stress-related. These include hypertension, high blood pressure, coronary thrombosis, heart attack, migraine, hay fever and allergies, asthma, peptic ulcers, constipation, colitis, rheumatoid arthritis, menstrual problems, nervous dyspepsia, flatulence and indigestion, hyperthyroidism (overactive thyroid gland), diabetes mellitus, skin disorders, tuberculosis, and finally depression.

CONTROLLING STRESS RESPONSE

We may not be able to alter the stress situations in life but we can alter how we cope. Natural healing and relaxation techniques (including reflexology), meditation, diet, and exercise can all help control or decrease the stress response and thereby lessen our susceptibility to stress-related diseases.

RIGHT
Stress has a resistance–lowering effect, making us more prone to disease.

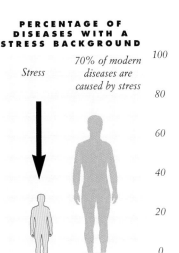

PERCENTAGE OF DISEASES WITH A STRESS BACKGROUND

Stress

70% of modern diseases are caused by stress

100

80

60

40

20

0

2 – LAURA NORMAN WITH THOMAS COWAN "FEET FIRST" P130   3 – ROBERT BECKER, M.D. AND GARY SELDON "THE BODY ELECTRIC" P292

HEART RATES

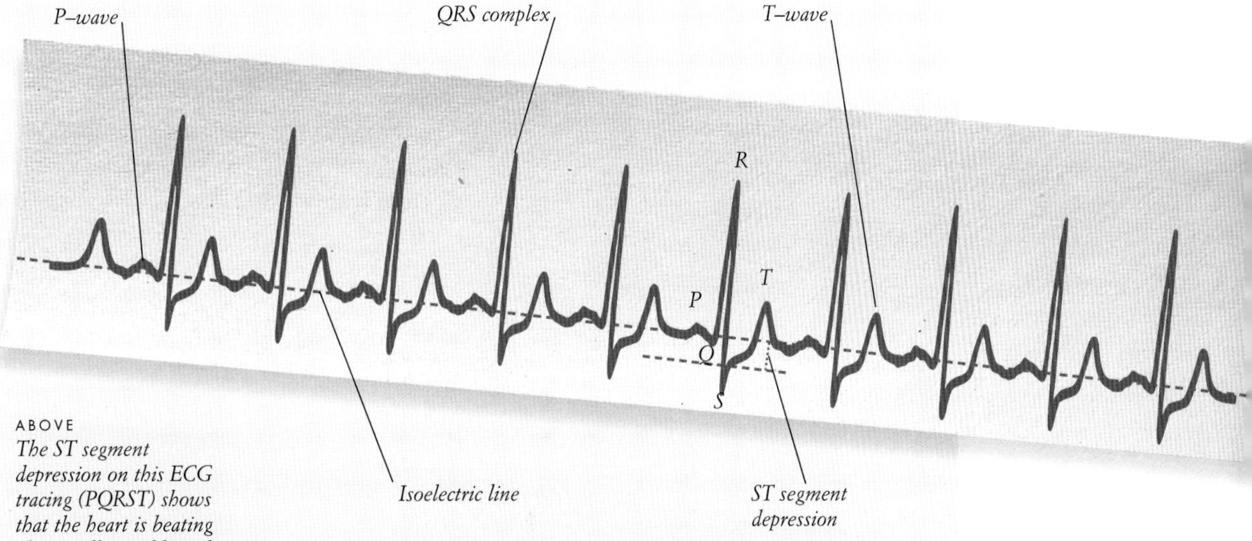

P–wave

QRS complex

T–wave

R

P

T

Q

S

ABOVE
The ST segment
depression on this ECG
tracing (PQRST) shows
that the heart is beating
abnormally quickly and
that the muscle is strained
by being short of blood.

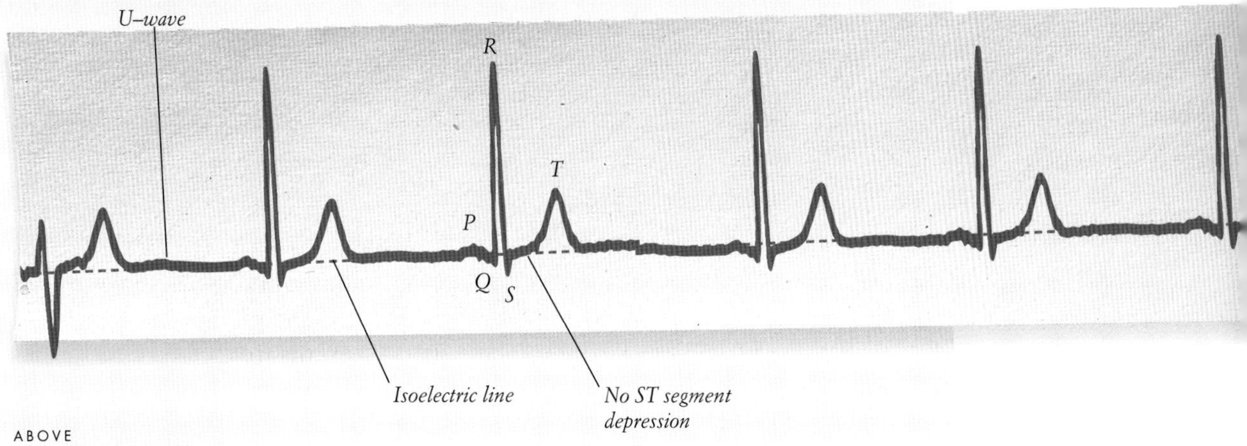

Isoelectric line

ST segment
depression

U–wave

R

P

T

Q S

Isoelectric line

No ST segment
depression

ABOVE
This ECG tracing shows a
normal heart. The rate is
normal and the PQRST
complexes are as well
(each PQRST complex
represents one heart beat).

LEFT

AN ELECTROCARDIOGRAM
(ECG) MEASURES THE
ELECTRICAL ACTIVITY OF
THE HEART AS IT BEATS
AND CAN HELP TO REVEAL
HOW MUCH STRESS THE
BODY IS EXPERIENCING.

25

3. UNDERSTANDING ENERGY

This book differs from the majority of reflexology books available today in that it incorporates the ancient Chinese concept of meridian therapy as an important and effective adjunct to reflexology.

RIGHT
Ancient systems of medicine recognize that the uninterrupted flow of energy around the body is the basis of health. The Chinese define the meridians as channels of energy, while the Hindu yogis, represented here, also point to seven energy centers, or chakras.

The "Vital Force"

Both zone therapy (to date, the primary basis of reflexology study) and meridian therapy are based on the premise that energy channels or pathways traverse throughout the body, linking organs and body parts. The efficacy of reflexology is believed to be the result of stimulating and revitalizing this energy flow. Thus it is necessary to have some concept of the fascinating phenomenon of energy.

Energy is the basis of all life and a vital factor in healing. As reflexologists, we are primarily concerned with internal body energy. A more comprehensive knowledge of this phenomenon will enhance our understanding of the interconnectedness of all things in the universe. This, in turn, will promote better comprehension of the holistic health philosophy – a philosophy of prime importance to anyone intending to study and practice reflexology.

All matter is made up of energy. The holistic health philosophy, of which reflexology is an important part, considers the human body as a dynamic energy system in a constant state of change. We are all an expression of energy and this energy permeates all living organisms. Because we cannot perceive energy with the naked eye, we find it difficult to comprehend, but this does not mean it does not exist.

In Chinese and Ayurvedic medicine, health is seen as the fluent and harmonious movement of energies at subtle levels. In the East this energy has various names. The Indian yogis call it *prana*; to the Tibetan lamas it is *lung-gom*. It is known as *sakia-tundra* or *ki* to the Japanese Shinto; and the Chinese call it *ch'i*. In the West it is loosely translated as "vital energy," "vital force," or "life force."

Yin and Yang are in equal proportions.

The constant flow of Yang into Yin and vice versa is represented by a curved line.

LEFT
The symbol of the Chinese yin and yang philosophy epitomizes the complementary nature of the two opposing elements.

WHAT IS CH'I

Ch'i is difficult to define. A good description is the following passage from *The Secret of the Golden Flower: A Chinese Book of Life:* "Heaven created water through One. If man attains the One he becomes alive; if he loses it he dies. But even if man lives in the energy (vital breath) he does not see the energy, just as fishes live in water but do not see the water. Man dies when he has not vital breath, just as fishes perish when deprived of water. If one guards this true energy, one can prolong the span of life and can apply the method of creating an immortal body."[1]

Vital energy represents some form of electricity. This does not mean it is electricity, but that its behavior, responses, and reactions indicate that many of the laws applying to electricity also apply to vital energy. According to Far Eastern tradition it circulates in the viscera, the flesh, and ultimately permeates every living cell and tissue. This energy is considered as having clearly distinct and established pathways, definite direction of flow, and characteristic behavior as well-defined as any other circulation such as blood and the vascular system.[2]

YIN AND YANG

A great deal of research into ch'i and meridians has been conducted in the last few decades, but access to this research is limited for Westerners since it is published in Chinese. Apparently, Chinese scientists are piecing together the fundamental characteristics of life energy. So far, they know it has four characteristics: electric, magnetic, infrared, and infrasonic. So many scientists in China are now concentrating their work in this field that a special branch of science – chiconology – has developed. The movement of energy is based on or is due to a relationship that

sets up two opposing fields; a "polarity." In Chinese philosophy this polarity relationship is called "yin and yang." Ted Kaptchuk says in his book *The Web That Has No Weaver,* "Yin-yang theory is based on the philosophical construct of two polar complements, called yin and yang. These complementary opposites are neither forces nor material entities. Nor are they mythical concepts that transcend rationality. Rather, they are convenient labels used to describe how things function in relation to each other and to the universe. They are used to explain the continuous process of natural change."[3]

In physical terms human beings can be reduced to a collection of electromagnetic fields. What we perceive as solid tissue is actually a mass of cells made up of chemical substances that are collections of atoms. Every atom consists of protons (positively charged), neutrons (no charge), and electrons (negatively charged). Electrons are more easily dislodged from atoms than protons so are the main carriers of electric charge.[4] Thus, at the atomic level the body is a mass of energy fields all influencing each other.

BELOW
A carbon atom is made up of a nucleus containing six protons and six neutrons, with six electrons rapidly orbiting the nucleus. Carbon is the basis of all living things.

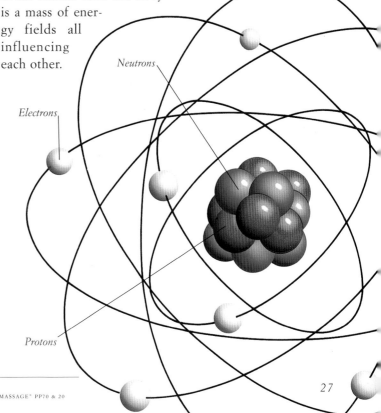

Neutrons

Electrons

Protons

1 – GEOFF PIKE "THE POWER OF CH'I" P9
2 – D. & J. LAWSON-WOOD "FIVE ELEMENTS OF ACUPUNCTURE AND CHINESE MASSAGE" PP70 & 20
3 – TED J. KAPTCHUK, O.M.D. "THE WEB THAT HAS NO WEAVER" P8
4 – ROBERT BECKER, M.D. AND GARY SELDON "THE BODY ELECTRIC" PP79–80

Science and the Life Force

The first "modern" scientific evidence of energy and the human body came from Dr. Harold Saxton Burr, Professor of Anatomy at Yale in the 1930s. He was convinced of the existence of "animal electricity" and developed apparatus to measure electrical potential even in minute organisms. He proved that humans, plants, and animals are surrounded by a life-field (L-field). Each produces an electric field that can be measured some distance away from the body and that mirrors and could possibly even control changes in the body. "Animals and plants," said Burr, "are essentially electric and show a change in voltage gradient associated with fundamental biological activity."[5]

Burr, the Editor of the *Yale Journal of Biology and Medicine*, published 28 papers outlining the bioelectric nature of menstruation, ovulation, sleep, growth, healing, and disease. He and his colleagues observed that changes in life-fields indicated changes taking place in the organisms producing these fields and used these to chart the course of health, predict illness, follow progress of healing in a wound, pinpoint movement of ovulation, diagnose psychic trauma, and measure the depth of hypnosis.[6] This energy field or "aura" can be perceived by "sensitive" people, and has been "proven" to exist by Kirlian photography – a technique that photographs the aura.

BELOW
All life is surrounded by its own energy field. These fields combine to contribute to a total field of electrical energy surrounding planet earth.

Kirlian researchers claim to be able to diagnose both the physical and emotional state of the body by the colors produced in the photograph and their intensity.

CONTROLLING CELL GROWTH WITH REFLEXOLOGY

Another Western physician who made an invaluable contribution to the use of electric energy in healing is Dr. Robert O. Becker. An orthopedic surgeon, he was interested in the possibility of electric current regenerating broken bones. Now patients can have small hearing aid batteries that produce a sustained negative charge implanted close to severe fractures that are reluctant to heal – with dramatic results. Becker was also interested in electricity as a factor in the overall control of cell differentiation and growth and proved that the right kind of current could inhibit infection, relieve pain, halt osteomyelitis, restore muscle control, repair intestinal ruptures, close holes in the heart, regenerate nerve cords, and replace lost parts in the brain.[7]

POLARITY THERAPY

Dr. Randolph Stone, who died in 1981 in India at the age of 91, combined Eastern and Western understanding to develop

5 – LYALL WATSON "BEYOND SUPERNATURE" PP92–7   6 – IBID   7 – IBID

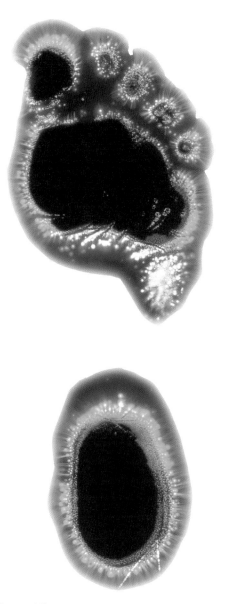

basis of life. Most people are beginning to accept that the physical world is part of a much larger whole – a whole that, unfortunately, most of us cannot physically perceive. We pick up only a fraction of what is going on around us, because our concepts of life are limited by our five senses.

From the barrage of electromagnetic waves in the environment living organisms select only those necessary for their survival. Although our brains are not geared to pick up TV waves, radio waves, and ultrasonic frequencies, we do not doubt their existence, so why should we doubt the existence of electrical energy merely because we can't see it?

ACHIEVING NATURAL BALANCE

Our bodies can benefit enormously from reflexology, and these benefits are maximized when treatment is carried out when our bodies are at their most receptive. This means that our lifestyle must be balanced, otherwise the benefits are soon dissipated. We may have to modify our diet, exercise, smoking, stress, and so on, but if we achieve the desired equilibrium, the rewards are great and we can gain the maximum potential benefit from reflexology treatment.

All life on earth is intricately interwoven with the natural rhythms and laws of the universe. Every organism regulates its metabolic activity in cycles attuned to the fluctuations of the earth, sun, and moon. So we humans are both directly and indirectly affected by various cosmic forces that are beyond our control. The optimum state for each individual is to live in complete harmony with nature and the surrounding environment. And it is the role of the reflexologist, working in accordance with the holistic philosophy, to help people to work toward and achieve this state of balance.

LEFT
Kirlian photography captures the energy field or "aura" surrounding the human body. The photograph shows the field clearly, because of high-energy interactions between the feet and applied electric field.

The earth's environment is composed of a whole host of electromagnetic waves that are not perceptible to the human being.

On earth, we humans can perceive only those parts of our world that we can experience through our five senses.

Polarity Therapy. A qualified osteopath and chiropractor, he came to define techniques for balancing the energy flow in human beings through his knowledge of Eastern wisdom, his understanding of the inner structure of the universe, and of the *gunas* described in Hindu literature. He developed, practiced, and taught Polarity Therapy in California and India with great success.[8]

THE BASIS OF LIFE

The West has finally discovered what the East has acknowledged for thousands of years – that electrical energy forms the

Energy in the Cosmos

BELOW
*The earth's
magnetic field
controls our
biological cycles.*

Our planet is a vibrant, pulsating mass of energy that lives and breathes in accordance with the natural laws of the universe. We as living organisms inhabiting this sphere are in turn electromagnetically intertwined with the energies of the earth. Our biological cycles are regulated by the earth's electromagnetic field; thus we are affected by changes in this field. The earth's field varies in response to the moon and the sun, so these too have an effect on us. To understand a little more of how these cosmic occurrences affect life, we will look briefly at the earth, sun, and moon.

EARTH

The earth's electromagnetic field is the result of interaction between the planet's molten nickel-iron core and the charged gas of the ionosphere.[9] This field is influenced by changes in lunar and solar events and it has a profound effect on life on the planet.

How are we as human beings related to this? Over the years researchers have come up with some interesting information. First is that the earth's magnetic field fluctuates between 8 and 16 times each second – the same as the prominent rhythm of our brain.[10] Also, the frequency of the micropulsations of the field is the prime timer of our biological cycles. Studies of the pineal gland have proved this statement. The pineal gland, which is situated in the center of the cranium, produces melatonin and seratonin, two neuro-hormones that (among many other functions) directly control all the biocycles. Small changes in magnetic fields influence the pineal gland – increasing or decreasing production of melatonin and seratonin.[11]

The reason for this could be magnetic attraction. Magnetic deposits have been discovered close to the pineal and pituitary glands in the sinuses of the ethmoid bone, the spongy bone in the center of the head behind the nose and between the eyes. It is possible that these deposits transmit the bio-cycle timing cues from the earth field's micropulsations to the pineal gland.[12]

To further illustrate the point, it has been proved that the L-fields described by Harold Saxton Burr register changes in response to sunlight, darkness, cycles of the moon, magnetic storms, and sunspots. This was discovered by testing the fields of trees – an excellent "subject" since they live to a great age and do not move around, so can be attached to equipment for extended periods. The fact that extraterrestrial forces have such a profound impact on the L-fields of trees indicates that they would probably have a more pronounced impact on the complex L-fields of humans.[13]

*Cerebrum controls
memory and
conscious thought.*

RIGHT
*The human brain
is thought to be
stimulated by
fluctuations in the
earth's magnetic
field. This brain
scan was obtained
by a technique
that detects
the magnetic
variations of parts
of the brain, called
magnetic resonance
imaging.*

*Brainstem controls heart rate,
blood pressure, breathing,
and unconsciousness.*

9 – ROBERT BECKER, M.D. AND GARY SELDON "THE BODY ELECTRIC" P247   10 – LYALL WATSON "GIFTS OF UNKNOWN THINGS" P105
11 – BECKER P249   12 – *IBID* P255   13 – HAROLD SAXTON BURR "BLUEPRINT FOR IMMORTALITY" P14

SUN

Energy for all the life on earth depends upon the sun. But this solar energy is not always positive. Human body functions are subject to some fairly extreme responses to sun-induced changes in the earth's magnetic field. One of the most disruptive effects of the sun is sunspot activity. This occurs in 11-year cycles and can be equated with nuclear explosions on the face of the sun, which emit a barrage of electromagnetic vibrations that bombard the earth. These solar disturbances can be related to major events on earth and have been known to coincide with social problems, with wars and epidemics. Sunspot activity was actually occurring at the time of the Black Death in England, the great plagues, diptheria and cholera outbreaks in Europe, the Russian typhus and smallpox epidemics.[14] The last six peaks of the 11-year sunspot cycles have coincided with major flu epidemics.

Dr. Robert Becker discovered correlations between disturbances in the earth's field caused by magnetic storms on the sun emitting "cosmic rays" and the rate of psychiatric admissions. He found that significantly more people were signed in to psychiatric services just after magnetic disturbances than when the earth's magnetic field was stable. He also found a similar influence on schizophrenic patients who exhibited behavior changes one or two days after cosmic ray decreases, due to low-energy cosmic ray flares from the sun that produce strong disruptions in the earth's magnetic field one or two days after the magnetic storms.[15]

MOON

The moon, too, has a profound influence on us. The earth attracts the moon strongly enough to hold it in the earth's orbit – and all bodies of water on the earth, both large and small, are affected by the moon. Because the human body is made up of approximately 75 percent water, it is obvious that humans too would be directly affected by the moon.

The moon affects conception and optimizes fertility levels. The average length of the menstrual cycle is almost identical to the time between two full moons. In some places the moon is referred to as "the great midwife."

The connection between the moon and madness has long been acknowledged – as is implied by the term "lunacy." Researchers at the American Institute of Climatology have investigated and published a report on the effect of a full moon on human behavior. The report records that crimes with strong psychotic motivation, such as arson, kleptomania, destructive driving, and homicidal alcoholism all show marked peaks at times when the moon is full.[16]

nspot

ABOVE
Sunspot activity affects the brain's magnetic responses. Sunspots, dark patches on the disk of the sun, are seen here just before the maximum in the 11-year cycle.

LEFT
The sun's energy can induce fluctuations in the earth's magnetic field.

ABOVE
The moon affects human fertility levels, crime levels, and is believed to be one of the causes of lunacy.

Artificial Energy

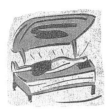

SUNBED
Ultraviolet rays

The earth's electromagnetic activity obviously has profound effects on life. So what of the effects of artificial energies? We have radically distorted our electromagnetic environment in the few decades since World War II. We are now completely surrounded by a sea of strange energies – the consequences of which we are only now beginning to discover.

Modern life revolves around electronic gizmos and gadgets. In the Western world, few homes or offices could function without a generous supply of "equipment": radios, televisions, computers, digital watches, microwave ovens, stereos, electronic locking systems, refrigerators, ovens, telephones, radar, electric trains, CB radios, electric blankets, and antitheft devices. Before the advent of electricity, radio, telephones, and other electronic "advances", the earth was quiet, and all organisms were regulated by the natural influences of the earth and nature.

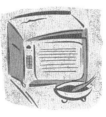

MICROWAVE
Microwaves

Today the world is a network of abnormal fields – the radio waves around us alone are now 100 to 200 million times the natural level reaching us from the sun.[17] These manufactured fields are producing abnormalities in both human and animal responses.

ELECTROMAGNETIC RADIATION

Electromagnetic radiation (EMR) encompasses an enormous range of frequencies – gamma rays, X-rays, ultraviolet wavelengths, infrared waves, microwaves (those we've harnessed for communication), and radio waves, which are broken down from extremely high to extremely low frequencies. It is extremely low frequen-

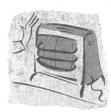

ELECTRIC FIRE
Infrared rays

cies (ELF) that seem most damaging to human health.[18]

Subliminal activation of the stress response is one of the most significant effects electromagnetic frequencies and nonionizing radiation have on life, but it is not the only one. These unfamiliar energies produce changes in nearly every bodily function so far studied.

In Russian research on rats, administration of steady

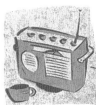

RADIO
Radio waves

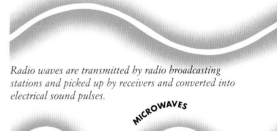

Radio waves are transmitted by radio broadcasting stations and picked up by receivers and converted into electrical sound pulses.

MICROWAVES

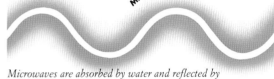

Microwaves are absorbed by water and reflected by metal. Microwave ovens heat food quickly because microwaves heat the water content by internal energy.

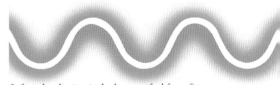

Infrared radiation is the heat we feel from fires or ovens and the sun. Anything warm gives off infrared radiation, and special cameras and film can detect this.

ULTRAVIOLET

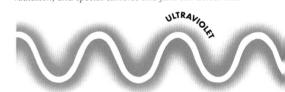

Ultraviolet rays from the sun are harmful to the human body, but ultraviolet light is also used to kill bacteria in milk.

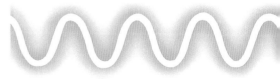

X-rays are used to photograph the inside of the human body. Most of the X-rays pass through the body, but some are absorbed by flesh and bone.

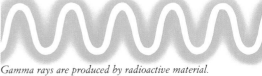

Gamma rays are produced by radioactive material. They are very dangerous to unprotected humans.

17 – BECKER P275 18 – *IBID* P272

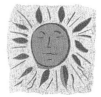

NUCLEAR REACTION
Gamma rays

magnetic fields caused cell death in the brain and generalized stress reaction marked by large amounts of cortisone in the bloodstream. This is a "slow" stress response evidencing prolonged stress, not the usual "fight-or-flight" response that is generated by adrenalin. Cortisone levels in four monkeys that had been exposed to a magnetic field for four hours a day showed stress response for six days when it subsided. This suggested adaption to the field – but this tolerance of continued stress is illusory.

Dr. Hans Selye, in his pioneering life- work on stress, explains that, initially, stress activates the hormonal and/or immune system to a higher than normal level, enabling the animal to escape danger or combat disease. If the stress continues, hormone levels and immune reactivity gradually decline to normal. However, if the stressful condition persists, hormone and immune levels decline further, well below normal. In medical terms stress decompensation has set in and the animal is now more susceptible to other stressors, including malignant growth and infectious diseases.[19]

SUN
Ultraviolet/infrared rays

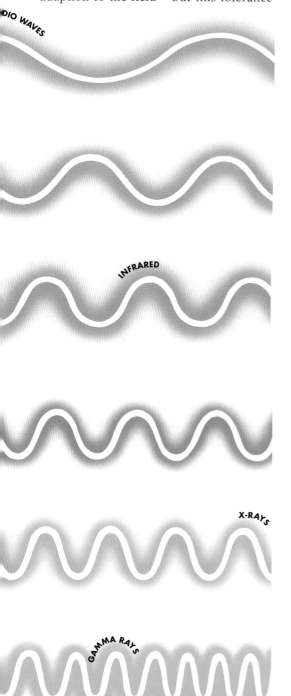

DIO WAVES

INFRARED

X-RAYS

GAMMA RAYS

ELECTROPOLLUTION

Most people are subject to extremely high daily exposure to so-called electropollution, particularly in cities that are subject to a whole spectrum of frequencies from ELF to microwave. The greatest danger lies in uncontrolled exposure to large amounts of electromagnetic radiation at many overlapping frequencies.[20] All cities, by their very nature as electrical centers, are jungles of interpenetrating fields and radiation that completely drown out the earth's background throb.[21] All life pulsates in time to the earth but the natural rhythms have now been overwhelmed by artificial fields, which can have drastic repercussions in all organisms.

So, how can we ever achieve health when we're being bombarded by an enemy we cannot perceive? We may have a role to play in dealing with the root cause of these conditions, but we should also remember that the correct effort to strengthen our own energy fields and state of health will increase our ability to cope with the additional stresses of electropollution. This is precisely where reflexology can help.

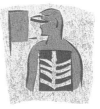

X-RAY MACHINE
X-rays

19 – BECKER P277   20 – IBID P313   21 – IBID P327

LEARNING TO RELAX

LEARNING TO RELAX IS
ONE OF THE MOST
POWERFUL ANTIDOTES
TO OUR STRESS-
INDUCED EXISTENCE.
MANY PEOPLE ARE
NOW TURNING TO
THERAPIES THAT OFFER
SAFE METHODS OF
INDUCING DEEP
RELAXATION, SUCH AS
REFLEXOLOGY AND
YOGA.

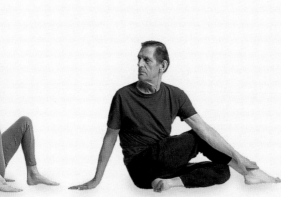

Gentle stretching exercises teach us how to relax the tension in our muscles.

More advanced stretches can aid digestion and make the spine more supple.

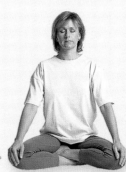

This classic posture is ideal for meditation, allowing the body to remain stable, the blood to circulate freely in the spine, and breathing to become deep and free.

LEFT
A relaxed body allows tension to fall away and the mind to be at peace.

Energy and a Healthy Diet

Few can honestly say they enjoy vibrant, boundless health, free from niggling aches, pains, allergies, and mood swings. In place of the dynamic energy that is our birthright, we have been conditioned to accept health as simply the absence of disease. Western nations spend millions on caring for the sick, and thousands of work-hours are lost every year through minor illnesses and impaired performance. Much of this needless suffering and expense could be alleviated if just a fraction of the money spent on remedial health was channeled into education on diet, nutrition, and prevention.

The one area of our lives over which most of us have total control is diet. It is also probably the most important factor in the maintenance of health and can be the greatest villain in the development of disease. The human body is constructed from the food we eat. Because we are constructed of energy fields, we are dependent on the energies we absorb from food. We should therefore eat foods compatible with our electrical energy needs that will stimulate rather than obstruct the free flow of energy in the body.

In the modern world an alarming amount of food is "dead." Pesticides, fertilizers, irradiation, and chemical additives serve to deplete the natural energy in food thereby depriving us of the vitality required to construct a healthy body. The increasing pressures of modern life also cause disruptions in the energy flow. Vitamins, minerals, proteins, fats, and carbohydrates are of no value if they cannot be assimilated because our bodies are themselves out of balance.

We know energy circulates throughout the body, influencing all the organs and body parts. Organs rely on correct energy circulation for correct functioning. Insufficient or depleted energy could damage the organs, and damaged organs will, in turn, interfere with the normal circulation of energy throughout the rest of the body.

One can equate this energy with a fire. Fire is vibrant, active, and dynamic. In order to burn brightly, a fire needs high-quality wood. Low-quality wood burns badly and does not generate sufficient heat, thus more wood is constantly required to feed the deficient flame.

Relating this to the body, if the vital energy symbolizes a fire, the wood can be equated with food. A body sustained on depleted junk food does not receive the necessary vitamins and minerals to function efficiently. As a result, the brain sends out messages for more nourishment. This craving is often dealt with by the consumption of caffeine, alcohol, and sugar-laden drinks. This is the equivalent of putting gasoline on the fire. A short sharp burst of instant energy is provided, but this is short-lived and suffers rapid burn-out. Then more "gasoline" is required to boost the flame again. This process cannot be maintained indefinitely without the body suffering for it. The fire needs to be sustained with the correct nourishment in order to burn steadily, strongly, and continuously. Only then can it create the energy necessary for a healthy body and mind.

LEFT
Store shelves today are laden with vitamin and mineral supplements, but these can only be absorbed into our systems if natural energy is allowed to flow freely around our bodies – a healthy diet is the best starting point.

THE EFFECTS
OF INCORRECT DIET

Depleted or stimulating food and drink also inflict stress on the body. Some form of reaction to this stress is inevitable. Physical manifestations will become apparent in the body systems, depending on where a person's particular weaknesses lie. Many health problems – heart disease, arthritis, kidney failure, gall bladder disorders, cancer, and hyperactivity – can be related to incorrect diet. More disturbing and less frequently acknowledged are the possible links between poor nutrition and behavior problems, aggression, and learning difficulties.

Many types of food on the market today should be labeled "toxic." Refined carbohydrates are classified as "susceptibility agents" (oversupply encourages disease). Since refined carbohydrates are grossly lacking in vitamins, minerals, essential fats, and protein, these foodstuffs are quite correctly labeled "empty calories." This group embraces table sugar, many precooked breakfast cereals, white flour, white (polished) rice, all highly sweetened foods (desserts, sweetened beverages, etc.), and both sweetened and unsweetened baked goods made from white wheat flour.

Many of the foods that we consume today have been processed in some way. Food processing has two major effects. First, it often changes and reverses the sodium/potassium ratio in foods. In the natural state most fruits and vegetables contain high levels of potassium and low levels of sodium. The body is good at conserving sodium and therefore requires very little; in contrast it is bad at conserving potassium and loses this vital element with alarming ease. Therefore a high potassium and low sodium diet is necessary. The second major effect of food processing is a reduction in the vitamin content of food, in some cases by a factor of ten times and in most cases by at least half. It is, therefore, possible to become vitamin deficient in the midst of plenty.[22]

RIGHT
INTAKE OF FOOD INTO THE BODY CAN BE EQUATED TO PUTTING FUEL ON A FIRE, WHERE THE FUEL IS FOOD AND THE FIRE IS ENERGY.

Sweet cakes and chocolate cookies have a high saturated fat and sugar content.

Fudge and sugar contain unnecessary calories.

White rice is refined and, therefore, has a reduced fiber content.

Hamburgers are high in cholesterol and fat.

Potato chips and french fried potatoes fried in oil are high in saturated fat.

White bread contains refined white flour, a source of "empty" calories.

INEFFICIENT ENERGY PRODUCTION

The resulting energy levels are inconsistent and the body suffers.

The body demands more intakes of food that give only short bursts of energy.

HOURS

Junk food represents poor burning body fuel, giving insufficient nourishment.

22 – DR. GEORGE LEWITH AND DR. JULIAN KENYON "CLINICAL ECOLOGY" P63

Fresh fruit such as grapes and oranges satisfy a craving for something sweet, but are also high in Vitamin C.

Brown pasta and wholemeal bread contain unrefined flour.

Bananas have a high fiber and potassium content.

Nuts contain protein – a good substitute for red meat.

Eat apples to obtain vitamins and fiber.

Lentils contain protein.

Oily fish such as herring are a good and nourishing source of protein and naturally unsaturated fat.

Brown rice is unrefined, retaining natural goodness and fiber.

Fresh vegetables contain most of the vitamins and minerals needed by the body for healthy growth.

EFFICIENT ENERGY PRODUCTION

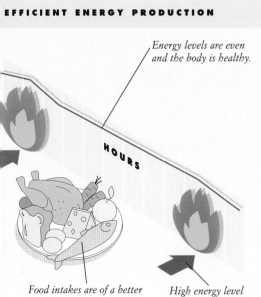

Energy levels are even and the body is healthy.

HOURS

Food intakes are of a better quality and so less frequent.

High energy level food burns strongly.

CHEMICAL CONTAMINATION

In addition to refined food we are also subjected to gross chemical contamination, which is harmful and can cause multiple sensitivities among other things. Contamination occurs in two main areas: the first is herbicide, pesticide, or weed-killer residues on fruit and vegetables and the presence of traces of synthetic hormones and antibiotics in meat. The second is the addition of chemicals to foods in order to improve their appearance and therefore saleability.

In one year the average person breathes in almost an ounce of solid pollution, eats 12lb. of food additives, has a gallon of herbicides and pesticides sprayed on the fruits and vegetables he or she eats, and receives nitrates and hormones from both water and food. No less than 6,000 new chemicals have been introduced into our food, homes, and the world around us in the last decade. Although we are equipped with mechanisms for detoxifying harmful substances, for many of us these mechanisms are becoming overloaded. When the total burden of pollutants exceeds our ability to detoxify, these substances are integrated into bone, fat, brain, and other tissues. The effects of pollution are cumulative.[23]

THE EFFECTS OF POLLUTION

Disease associated with high levels of pollutants include all forms of arthritis, allergies, candidiasis, ME, repeated infections, hyperactivity, high blood pressure, asthma, acne, eczema, and schizophrenia. Minor symptoms associated with an increased body burden of pollutants include lethargy, drowsiness, mood swings, inability to concentrate, intolerance of fat or alcohol, poor skin, body odor, headaches, nausea, skin rashes, frequent infections, and multiple allergies. All of these can occur for other reasons but are more likely to occur in those who are not adequately nourished.[24]

LEFT
A good diet is essential for a healthy body. The left side of the plate contains foods that should be labeled as "toxic" and may cause behavior problems in those who consume them. The right side of the plate shows a selection of the foods you should eat for a healthy lifestyle.

23 – PATRICK HOLFORD "POLLUTION PROTECTION" IN "HERE'S HEALTH" MAGAZINE, AUGUST 1989, P13   24 – IBID P13

How Reflexology Revitalizes Energy

As we have seen, the body is a dynamic energy field. The Chinese discovered that this energy – ch'i – circulates along 12 meridian pathways within the body. (This aspect is discussed in more depth in Part 2, page 62.) The six main meridians that penetrate the major organs of the body are found in the feet – specifically in the toes. Massaging the meridian pathways in the feet helps clear blockages along the meridians and encourages the vital body energy to flow.

ELECTRICAL IMPULSES

The theory that some form of energy animates the body is now more widely acknowledged by many scientists and medical practitioners. And the belief that this energy is revitalized through reflexology treatment is expounded by many modern reflexologists.

Ann Gillanders, for example, says: "The body is based on an electrical circuit and like normal circuits has negative and positive poles. Reflexology is a method of contacting the electrical centres in the body and has been used for centuries to create a smooth flow of vibratory energy through the body by contacting various points in the feet which relate to various organs, glands and cells."[25]

Doreen Bayley, has this to say: "There is, I believe, an electrical impulse trig-

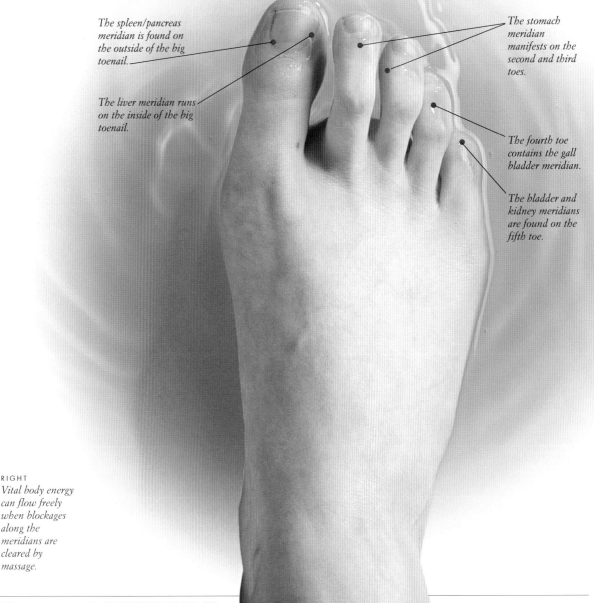

The spleen/pancreas meridian is found on the outside of the big toenail.

The liver meridian runs on the inside of the big toenail.

The stomach meridian manifests on the second and third toes.

The fourth toe contains the gall bladder meridian.

The bladder and kidney meridians are found on the fifth toe.

RIGHT
Vital body energy can flow freely when blockages along the meridians are cleared by massage.

25 – GILLANDERS "REFLEXOLOGY – THE ANCIENT ANSWER TO MODERN AILMENTS" P25

IMPEDED AND UNIMPEDED ENERGY FLOW

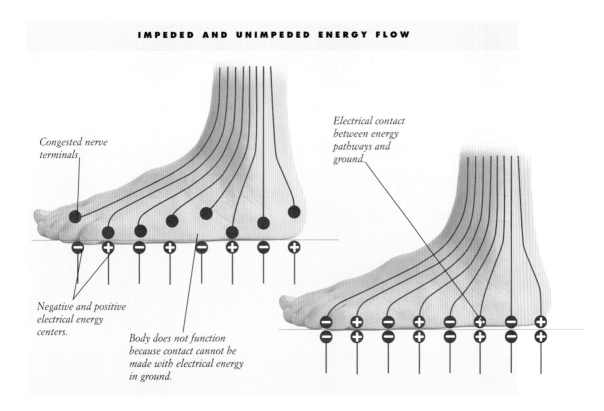

Congested nerve terminals.

Electrical contact between energy pathways and ground.

Negative and positive electrical energy centers.

Body does not function because contact cannot be made with electrical energy in ground.

gered off by pressure massage on a tender reflex and there is a subtle flow which brings that remarkable return of vitality to the patient even while receiving treatment. I believe that the electrical impulse acts on the body in the same way that the stimulus of light acts on the retina of the eye. It has been proven that the action of the full spectrum of light on the retina of the eye, in which are embedded the endings of the optic nerve, produces an electrical impulse which is carried to the hypothalamus, from whence it passes down to the pituitary gland, which passes down to the lesser glands, thereby activating all the functions of the body. It is my belief that the work upon the reflexes produces similar results."[26]

Eunice Ingham, the "Mother of Modern Reflexology," states: "The nerves of our body may be likened to an electrical system. It will be our ability to make normal contact with the electricity in the ground, through our feet and from the elements or atmosphere surrounding us, that will determine the degree of power we are able to manifest in proper functioning of the glands. Trying to get a

normal contact when there is congestion in these nerve terminals in the feet is like trying to put a plug into a defective fixture."[27]

OPENING THE PATHWAYS

For the human organism to function at optimum capacity, energy must flow unimpeded and the yin and yang energy currents must complement each other. Reflexology opens up the energy pathways, energizing the physical, emotional, and mental aspects of the client. The specific techniques for applying pressure to the feet create channels for healing energy to circulate to all parts of the body. When the body is "out of balance" it is not functioning efficiently. Reflexology helps return the body to a dynamic state of balance. When the reflexes on the feet are stimulated, an involuntary response is elicited in organs and glands connected by energy pathways or meridians to these specific reflexes. A chain reaction is then set in motion causing physiological changes to occur throughout all the sytems of the body.

ABOVE
If our nerve terminals are congested, the flow of energy between the earth and our bodies is impeded. Reflexology unblocks the pathways allowing energy to flow freely.

26 – ANDREW STANWAY, M.B. M.R.C.P. "ALTERNATIVE MEDICINE" P36   27 – GEOFF PIKE "THE POWER OF CH'I" P9

4. HOW CAN REFLEXOLOGY HELP?

We have already seen how reflexology can be used to alleviate the effects of stress, induce relaxation, revitalize the body's energy and rebalance its whole system. In this chapter we look more closely at further specific areas of application.

The Nervous System

The nervous system is the body's "electrical system," and it is the most complex system in the body. Without a nerve supply the organs of the body could not function. Every part of the body is operated by messages carried back and forth along neural pathways. The nervous system is divided into three parts: the central nervous system, the peripheral nervous system, and the autonomic nervous system. It is believed that nerve impulses initiated through pressure on the reflexes of the feet may be connected to the autonomic nervous system.

The autonomic nervous system controls the involuntary action of internal organs, muscles, and glands. As we have seen there are two parts to the system – the sympathetic and parasympathetic. These parts have opposing effects on the body. They both send out weak impulses to the organs and glands to maintain normal activity. However, in stressful situations, the sympathetic impulses become stronger and the organs and glands react to the situation. The parasympathetic system takes over when the stress has passed and returns the body functions to normal.

STIMULATING THE REFLEXES

Many reflexologists believe that stimulating the reflex areas of the feet has an effect on the internal organs via a simple reflex action. A reflex is an unconscious or involuntary response to a stimulus. Some reflex actions are quite common and simple, such as the pupil of the eye reacting to light, or the jerk of the leg

Bra*

Spinal cord

Cervical nerves supply neck, shoulders, and arms.

Thoracic nerves supply trunk and arms.

Lumbar nerves supply legs and lower back.

Sacral nerves supply legs and genitals.

RIGHT
The nervous system makes the body's organs function correctly. Pressure on the feet reflexes stimulates the autonomic nervous system.

REFLEX ACTION

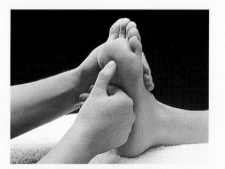

Reflexologist applies stimulus, here to the heart reflex on the left foot.

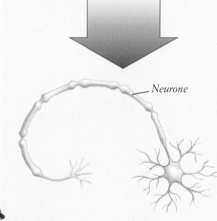

Neurone

Electrochemical nerve impulse is activated and is conducted to the central nervous system by a sensory neurone.

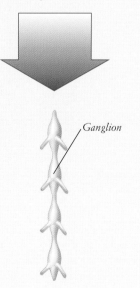

Ganglion

The message, received by the ganglion, is transmitted via a motor neurone, which causes a response.

when the knee is tapped. For a reflex action to occur there must first be a stimulus. In the case of reflexology, the stimulus is provided when pressure is applied to the reflex area of the feet. This activates an electrochemical nerve impulse that is conducted to the central nervous system via a sensory (afferent) neurone. This message is received by the ganglion and the message is then transmitted via a motor (efferent) neurone, which then causes a response.

The autonomic nervous system does not work apart from the rest of the nervous system. A loud noise perceived by the sensory system can speed up the beating of the heart, thereby influencing the entire circulatory system. A chronic state of worry, anxiety, fear, or excitement involving a voluntary part of the nervous system will often result in pathological conditions involving the autonomic part of the nervous system.[1]

NEURAL PATHWAYS

The neural pathways are both living tissue and electrical channels and can be impinged upon or polluted by many factors. When neural pathways are impaired nerve function is impeded, messages are delivered slowly and unreliably, and body processes operate at less than optimum levels. Reflexology, by stimulating the thousands of nerve endings in the feet, encourages an opening and clearing of neural pathways.

LEFT
Reflexology is believed to stimulate internal organs of the body by a simple reflex action.

The Circulation

One of Eunice Ingham's favorite sayings was "Circulation is life. Stagnation is death." Every practitioner acknowledges the importance of good circulation. If the smallest fraction of circulation is cut off from one or more parts of the body, the effects soon become evident in a variety of aches and pains. All the tissues of the body depend on an adequate blood supply to function correctly, and the application of reflexology benefits the body circulation.

More than 1,000 times a day blood circulates in one direction through the body's 60,000-mile network of veins and arteries. About 24,000 gallons of blood pass through the heart daily. Red blood cells carry oxygen around the body during their 120-day lifespan. White blood cells fight disease by digesting germs.

Blood carries oxygen and nutrients to the cell and removes waste products and toxins. During this process, blood vessels contract and relax, so their resilience is most important for correct functioning. Stress and tension tighten up the cardiovascular system and restrict blood flow. Circulation becomes sluggish, causing high and low blood pressure.

The increased state of relaxation facilitated by reflexology allows all the body systems – including the excretory systems – to function efficiently by allowing them to eliminate toxins and impurities thoroughly. By reducing stress and tension, reflexology allows the cardiovascular vessels to conduct the flow of blood naturally and easily.

Circulatory factors are influenced by the pressure applied in reflexology. The effects of reflexology on blood pressure have been proven in a blood pressure study at the California Police Olympics, where reflexologists participated in "demonstration" booths during the games held in 1987. A small informal blood pressure study was conducted by the Sacramento Valley Reflexology Association. It was found that reflexology normalized (either brought it up or down, as needed) the systolic pressure in 75 percent and normalized the diastolic pressure in 61 percent of those cases that were studied.[2]

CRYSTAL DEPOSITS

Grainy crystal deposits, which cause pain during treatment, may be felt in the nerve endings of the feet. These are believed to be calcium deposits that have settled beneath the skin surface at the nerve endings. Excess acidity in the bloodstream increases calcium deposits in the nerve endings of any organ in the body. These deposits develop into acid crystals that can impede normal blood circulation.

The feet are a prime target of these congestions because of the abundance of nerve endings present here and the fact that feet are usually restricted in shoes preventing the natural movement of the foot. Thus the normal nerve and blood supply to the feet is slowed down. The feet are also at the end point of circulation, and blood has to be circulated back up against the force of gravity. Congestion will impede this function, and toxins will tend to stagnate in the feet. These crystals can be broken down by reflexology massage and the residue removed by the blood circulation.

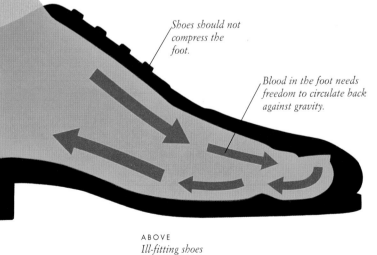

Shoes should not compress the foot.

Blood in the foot needs freedom to circulate back against gravity.

ABOVE
Ill-fitting shoes may restrict the free circulation of blood around the foot.

The Endocrine System

Hypothalamus controls the pituitary gland. Pituitary glands secretes growth hormone and antidiuretic hormones regulating body's water level.

Thyroid gland secretes thyroid hormone essential for life.

Veins

Adrenal glands secrete adrenaline and noradrenaline, enabling the body to cope with stress.

Pancreas secretes insulin maintaining the body's blood sugar level.

Ovaries (and testes in men) secrete the reproductive hormones of estrogen, progesterone, and testosterone.

Uterus

If the nerves are considered the "electrical" system of the body, then the endocrine glands are the "chemical" system. The endocrine system is an intricate network of glands that secrete hormones directly into the blood. Hormones are extremely powerful chemical substances. If any one of the seven principal glands is out of order, hormone secretion will be disrupted and, in consequence, the whole body thrown off balance.

The pancreas provides an excellent example. One of its main functions is to maintain the balance of glucose or blood sugar. The hormone insulin activates the body cells to take up the glucose from the blood. The body cells or tissues break this glucose down into carbon dioxide and water to produce energy and it is stored by the liver as glycogen.

Without insulin, the glucose is not consumed or is stored incorrectly. It accumulates in the blood causing diabetes. When insulin removes glucose from the blood by increased combustion, the storage of glycogen is increased at the expense of the blood. Low blood sugar (hypoglycemia) is the result. The balance has been disrupted.[3]

GLAND FUNCTION

Every tissue and organ in the body is controlled by complex chemical interaction. The hormones secreted by the anterior part of the pituitary gland, often referred to as the master gland of the body, are under the influence of the hypothalamus. Nerves connect the thymus and spleen directly to the hypothalamus, which affects the immune system. In essence, the brain controls the immune system.[4]

Thoughts and emotions are affected by the glands, and personality is determined by gland function. If gland function is harmonious, one will have a positive happy outlook; disharmonious function will cause a depressive outlook. Reflexology, by stimulating the electrical energy, has a subsidiary effect on the chemical energy.

LEFT
The endocrine system is the body's chemical system secreting hormones into the blood.

Pain Control

A number of chemical changes take place in the body during reflexology treatment. One such change deals with the sedation of pain. The body produces its own painkillers, known as endorphins, which are five to ten times more powerful than morphine. Endorphins are produced by the pituitary gland and can inhibit the transmission of pain signals through the spinal cord.

Studies have revealed that pain signals travel along the nerve pathways to the dorsal horn of the spinal cord, beginning a complicated reflex action. From the spinal cord the impulse is relayed to the thalamus, where the sensations of heat, cold, pain, and touch are recognized. The thalamus forwards the impulse along to the cerebral cortex where the intensity and location of the pain is recognized. The brain then sends signals back through the spinal cord to release endorphins. However, according to the "gate control theory," the nervous system can respond to only a limited amount of sensory information at one time. When

RIGHT
Reflexology can stimulate the pituitary gland helping the body to produce more endorphins to reduce pain.

the system becomes overloaded it short-circuits, or closes a gate, reducing the amount of sensory information available for processing. The application of reflexology encourages the brain to produce more endorphins while the pressure also acts to confuse the body with too many sensations to respond to, forcing the body to close the "pain gates."[5] This interrupts the pain cycle, eases pain and helps the body to relax.[6]

RIGHT

REFLEXOLOGY ACTS IN TWO WAYS TO REDUCE PAIN: BY ENCOURAGING THE BODY TO PRODUCE ENDORPHINS AND BY INTERRUPTING THE PAIN CYCLE THROUGH THE APPLICATION OF PRESSURE.

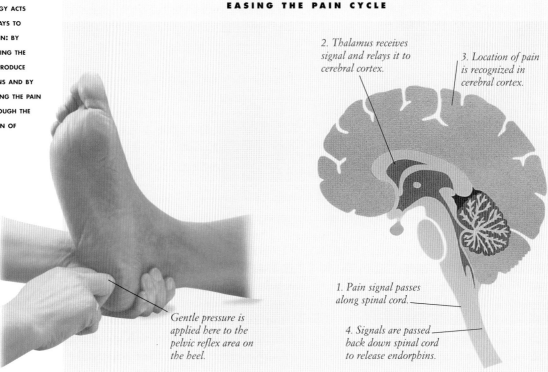

EASING THE PAIN CYCLE

2. Thalamus receives signal and relays it to cerebral cortex.

3. Location of pain is recognized in cerebral cortex.

1. Pain signal passes along spinal cord.

4. Signals are passed back down spinal cord to release endorphins.

Gentle pressure is applied here to the pelvic reflex area on the heel.

5 – ISSEL PP117-18   6 – IBID P77

Terminal Diseases

In cases of terminal illness such as cancer, multiple sclerosis, and Aids, reflexology may not be capable of removing the cause of the disease but it does make the patient more comfortable and the pain more bearable. It can significantly improve the patient's general condition, activate excretory organs, stimulate the respiratory system, and help the patient achieve better control of the bladder and bowels. Muscular spasms associated with multiple sclerosis may be reduced in severity and frequency, and the weakness of the whole body can often be improved. With Aids, reflexology can work on the immune system, helping to prolong life.

In our high-tech biomedical era, the possibility of miraculous cures and new technical developments is held out as a thread of hope to patients with terminal diseases, when common sense may dictate that such hope is deceptive. In the care of advanced diseases it may be more realistic – and, ultimately, more beneficial to the patient – to improve a person's quality of life on a day-to-day basis, and reflexology has an important part to play in this.

QUALITY OF LIFE

Reflexology has a significant role to play in enhancing the daily quality of life of patients with terminal diseases.

A gentle caring touch can be therapeutic.

Pain can be eased through gentle pressure.

occasional visits to a reflexologist as extra "maintenance" potentially can be of enormous benefit.

Preventive therapy is useful for people who have completed a course of treatment and want to avoid any problem reemerging, as well as for those who may not have any acute symptoms but realize the need for preventive action. Treatments at regular intervals can assist the body in maintaining a balanced state, and prevent the possibility of slight imbalances becoming troublesome.

Almost every person, however young or old, will enjoy and benefit from reflexology. It is instinctively more difficult to abuse the body once internal communication and attunement have been reestablished within the body.

The intervals between treatments will vary from person to person and may involve weeks or months. For best results, treatment should be applied in the correct manner by a trained therapist, but it can also be beneficial to work on certain reflexes oneself between sessions to act as a boost to the treatment.

Reflexology as Preventive Therapy

Health-threatening dangers lurk around every corner in our modern environment: polluted land, air, and water, contaminated food, contaminated environment. Add to this the stress of our day-to-day lives – bad diet, attitudes, and lifestyle – and we have a potentially lethal cocktail designed to encourage disease. Most people wait until disease rears its ugly head before seeking help, but it is infinitely more sensible to listen to the body's warning signals and take action early. In addition to caring for the body by eating more sensibly, exercising, and calming the mind and body with relaxation and also meditation techniques,

LEFT
Visiting your reflexologist for regular diaried appointments will help you to maintain your body in the balance arrived at through the therapy.

Reflexology Case Histories

All the case histories described here refer to real people whose conditions have been successfully treated with reflexology. The individual case histories cover a variety of ailments and conditions, but all show how regular reflexology treatment benefited each person's whole body and attitude to life.

RIGHT
A heavy workload resulted in a number of stress-related problems for this client.

FATIGUE

A 27-year-old physician found increasing fatigue made her long hours of work difficult to cope with. She felt lethargic, tired, and generally under the weather. An increase of 7lb. in weight, frequent sore throats, spots on the upper chest, forehead, nose, and around the mouth, and headaches accompanied the fatigue. Her sight had deteriorated over the past three years and she wore contact lenses occasionally but could not tolerate them for long. She was sensitive to smoke, suffered sinus problems, and flatulence. Sore breasts and candida appeared prior to her period. She was prone to mood swings, tension, and found her concentration poor. Her hands and her feet were cold and purple.

Following the first treatment she was in a bad mood for three days, headachy, and tired. Then her concentration improved, she felt more relaxed, lost 2lb., her throat, colic, flatulence, bowel movement, and sinus all improved. At the third treatment, her energy was "brilliant," she had lost another 2lb., and her mood had improved tremendously. She felt calm and relaxed, and could cope with her workload.

RIGHT
A special diet was insufficient to cure a client's psoriasis.

PSORIASIS

A 23-year-old man developed a problem with psoriasis when he was four years old. It now covered his chest, stomach, back, behind his ears, forehead, knees, elbows, and inner thighs. Two years previously it had been so severe he had gone on a special diet. This helped but he had to give it up because he lost too much weight. He had a poor appetite, was bloated after eating, had a stiff neck, and painful shoulder blades especially on waking, and his ears felt full and waxy. His eyes were weak and sensitive, being painful when he moved from light to dark, twitching and losing focus when reading. He also suffered extreme fluctuations in mood, headaches, and had a tendency to lethargy.

The second treatment saw him very tired, depressed, and out of breath, with little improvement in symptoms. But by the third treatment the psoriasis had visibly improved, as had his appetite and energy level. Although his eyes were still sensitive, the headaches were milder, and he felt calmer and happier. At the fifth treatment all the symptoms had improved. He had a four-month break and then 14 regular treatments by which time his skin was almost perfect, he had gained weight, was revitalized and had no aches and pains at all.

INSOMNIA

For ten years prior to seeking reflexology treatment, a 58-year-old man had suffered from disrupted sleep patterns – waking up every night and reading for a few hours in an attempt to tire his brain. Although his energy level was good, he was apt to doze off around lunchtime and in the evenings.

A tennis injury seven years before had resulted in a frozen shoulder for which he was on medication – osteopathic help had not solved the problem. Neck pressure caused terrible headaches over the eye area. Another sports injury resulted in torn knee ligaments, and therefore stiffness when walking down the stairs.

He had a fungal infection in a nail for seven to eight years for which he had taken medication, but the side-effects caused diarrhea so he discontinued the medication.

His eyesight was deteriorating and he had watering eyes and ringing in his ears. He was also a terrible worrier, fussy, and had difficulty in forming lasting relationships with other people.

At the second reflexology treatment he was far more relaxed. The noise in his ears had ceased, nighttime sleep patterns had improved, he was dozing off less often, his shoulder and neck were fine, no headaches, eyes had stopped watering, knees had improved and he was a lot less worried.

By the fifth treatment he was sleeping peacefully right through the night. His knees were fine, even when he played in a tennis tournament. He felt completely relaxed and fully revitalized.

LEFT
A keen tennis player sustained severe sports injuries that benefited from reflexology.

M.E.
(Chronic Fatigue Syndrome)

Up to two years prior to his first reflexology treatment, this 39-year-old man had enjoyed good health. He suddenly began to feel very ill, and experienced panic attacks and fainting spells. His white blood cell count was high and he had not been well since.

Nine months previously he had begun to experience giddiness when tilting his head, for which he was prescribed stabilizing tablets that only aggravated the situation. He felt more peculiar every day but another blood test revealed his white cell count had returned to normal. He

had great difficulty getting out of bed, and experienced almost continual weakness and exhaustion. Because of these symptoms he had been off work for six months. His chest, bladder, and stomach were weak and he often suffered from pins and needles in his left hand. Following numerous tests and a brain scan he was diagnosed as having Myalgic Encephalomyelitis (ME).

After the first reflexology treatment he felt tired and light-headed, but by the third treatment he felt much more optimistic and cheerful. He no longer felt he needed to sleep during the day. Over the course of treatment his health was up and down, but after 20 treatments he was sufficiently recovered to return to work. Although he still suffered some aches and pains, his concentration, memory, and energy level had improved, the main problematic symptoms had been eliminated and he felt he was once again able to cope.

LEFT
After six months absence from work due to ME this client sought reflexology treatment and was back at work after 20 treatments.

47

5. THE HISTORY OF REFLEXOLOGY

The roots of reflexology are embedded way back in ancient history when pressure therapies were recognized as preventive and therapeutic medicine. Exactly where and how it all began is somewhat elusive, but evidence indicates that therapeutic foot massage has been practiced throughout history by a variety of cultures.

Feet Facts

BELOW
Leonardo da Vinci made a comprehensive study of the structure of the human foot, calling it a masterpiece of engineering.

Feet have an illustrious and intriguing history. Anthropologists regard the foot as the definitive human physical trait. When the first anthropoid straightened up from a four-legged crouch approximately 50 million years ago, the feet, originally designed to carry one-quarter of the body weight each, had to adjust to carrying half each. The spinal column, originally an arch between forefeet and back feet, had to adapt to the upright position. The thumblike big toe then moved into the same plane as the other toes, and the heel dropped to rest on the ground to support the body weight more efficiently. Finally the arches evolved to contribute to our stride.[1] Leonardo da Vinci called the foot a masterpiece of engineering and a work of art. Considering the size of feet in relation to the body they support, the humble feet are nothing short of remarkable.

THE FOOT IN CULTURE

The best-known mythological reference is Achilles' heel. The story goes that while dipping Achilles in water to render him invulnerable, his mother held him by one heel. This small part of his anatomy that missed submersion was ultimately the cause of his demise. The term "Achilles' heel" is still commonly used today to refer to a person's weak spot.[2]

The Greek foot – a term derived from ancient mythology – originally referred to goddesses with longer second toes, which was symbolic of their male powers.[3] And virgin goddesses were always depicted covering their feet to protect their chastity since feet were considered extremely private parts. Revealing the feet was the equivalent of a blatant proposition.[4]

The Asian custom of foot kissing was a gesture of submission toward a person of lofty status like a pope or a saint. The removal of shoes at the threshold of holy places is observed by Buddhists, Hindus, and Muslims. This, too, appears in the Bible – when God said to Moses: "Put off thy shoes from thy feet, for the place whereon thou standest is holy ground."[5]

In Chinese cultures, a woman's foot was regarded as the ultimate sex symbol. To render the feet the most attractive parts of the anatomy and mold them into the desired shape, women's feet were bound. This prevented bones from developing in the usual way and stunted foot growth. This uncomfortable, unkind practice has fortunately been discontinued.[6]

1 – MICHELLE ARNOT "FOOT NOTES" PP8-9   2 – IBID P26   3 – IBID P21   4 – IBID Pxx   5 – IBID P28   6 – IBID P30

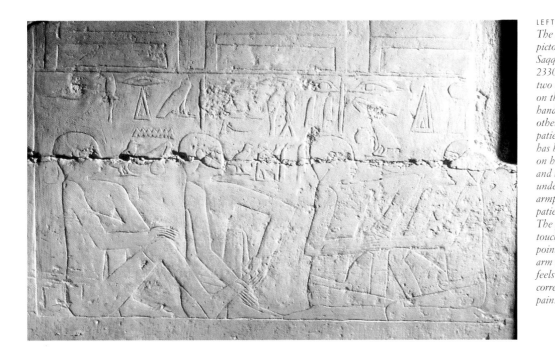

LEFT
The scene from a pictograph at Saqqara (2500-2330 B.C.)depicts two men working on the feet and hands of two other men. The patient on the left has his right hand on his right knee and his left hand under his right armpit. The other patient is opposite. The patient is touching the reflex point under his arm where he feels the corresponding pain.

The Roots of Reflexology

A widely held theory is that reflexology originated in China about 5,000 years ago. Many reputable reflexologists have stated their belief in this theory even though concrete proof is evasive. Egyptian and Babylonian cultures developed before Chinese culture, however, and Egypt contributed a valuable piece of historical evidence.

The oldest documentation depicting the practice of reflexology was unearthed in Egypt. This evidence, a pictograph dated around 2500–2330 B.C., was found in the tomb of an Egyptian physician, Ankmahor, at Saqqara. According to evidence found in the tomb, Ankmahor was considered to be a most influential person – second only to the king.

THE CHEROKEE NATIVE AMERICANS

Another theory claims that a form of reflex therapy was passed down to the Native Americans by the Incas. Again, no specific evidence supports this theory. However, the use of reflex pressure applied to the feet as a healing therapy has been practiced by the North American native peoples for generations. For centuries the Cherokee of North Carolina have acknowledged the importance of feet in maintaining physical, mental, and spiritual balance. The Bear Clan from this tribe who live in the hills of the Allehjanies can attest to this.

Jenny Wallace, a Cherokee from a Bear Clan, practices as a foot therapist today. In the tribe, she is known as a "moon maiden" – a title bestowed on a woman who, as a young girl, exhibits natural intuitive healing talents and is chosen by the tribe to develop these further. According to Wallace: "In my tribe working on the feet is a very important healing art and is part of a sacred ceremony that you don't have to be ill to take part in. The feet walk upon the earth and through this your spirit is connected to the universe. Our feet are our contact with the earth and the energies that flow through it."[7]

This knowledge of foot reflex therapy might have been lost to antiquity had it not been for inquiring medical minds of the late 19th and early 20th centuries. People intrigued by the concept of reflex therapy instigated a resurgence of interest in the study of reflexology. The study and development of reflex therapy by pioneering Europeans and enterprising Americans laid the foundations of reflexology as we know it today.

The Development of Zone Therapy

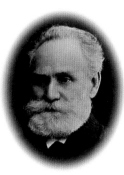

ABOVE
*Ivan Pavlov
developed the
theory of
conditioned
reflexes in 1870.*

BELOW
*The feet have
been divided into
zones for the
purposes of
pressure-therapy
in Europe since
the 14th century.
Dr. William
Fitzgerald divided
the feet into
ten longitudinal
zones in the
19th century.*

In Europe a form of reflexology was known and practiced as far back as the 14th century. According to Harry Bond Bressler in his book *Zone Therapy,* "Pressure therapy was well known in the middle countries of Europe and was practised by the working classes of those countries as well as by those who catered to the diseases of royalty and the upper class." Dr. Adamus and Dr. A'tatis wrote a book on the subject of zone therapy that was published in 1582.[8]

The scientific basis of reflex study had its roots in neurological studies conducted in the 1890s by Sir Henry Head of London. In 1898 he discovered zones on the skin that became hypersensitive to pressure when an organ connected by nerves to this skin region was diseased. After years of clinical research Sir Henry Head established what became known as "Head's Zones" or "zones of hyperalgesia."

RUSSIAN WORK

Russian work on reflexes began from a psychological point of view. The founder of Russian physiology Ivan Sechenov (who discovered the cerebral inhibition of spinal reflexes) published a paper in 1870 titled "Who Must Investigate the Problems of Psychology and How?" Psychologists under Vladimir Bekhterev, who founded St. Petersburg's Brain Institute, picked up the challenge and studied it through reflexes. At the same time Ivan Pavlov (1849–1936) read Sechenov's work and acknowledged that his book *Reflexes of the Brain* was the most important theoretical inspiration for his own work on conditioning. Pavlov developed the theory of conditioned reflexes – namely that there is a simple and direct relationship between a stimulus and a response. He found that practically any stimulus can act as a conditioning stimulus to produce a corresponding conditioned response.[9]

GERMAN TECHNIQUES

Today the Russians continue to pursue the study of reflexology from both the physiological and psychological point of view. They have scientifically tested the effect of reflex therapy on patients with a variety of problems and have found reflexology to be an effective complement to traditional medicine.[10]

At the same time, the Germans were also looking into the treatment of disease by massage. In the late 1890s and early 1900s massage techniques developed in Germany became known as "reflex massage." This was the first time that the benefits of massage techniques were specifically credited to reflex actions.

Dr. Alfons Cornelius was possibly the first to apply massage to "reflex zones." The story goes that in 1893 Cornelius suffered from an infection. In the course of his convalescence he received a daily massage. At the spa he noticed how effective the massages of one particular medical officer

8 – HARRY BOND BRESSLER "ZONE THERAPY" P29
9 – ISSEL PP30-31   10 – IBID P35

were. This man worked longer on areas he found painful. This concept inspired Cornelius. After examining himself, Cornelius instructed his masseur to work only on the painful areas. His pain quickly disappeared and in four weeks he completely recovered. This led him to pursue the use of pressure in his own medical practice. He published his manuscript "Druckpunkte" or "Pressure Points, The Origin and Significance" in 1902.[11]

Europeans went on to expand on the research initiated by the abovementioned people. But credit for putting modern reflexology on the map must go to a number of Americans.

THE AMERICAN INFLUENCE

Dr. William Fitzgerald, commonly known as the founder of zone therapy, was born in Connecticut, in 1872. He graduated in medicine from the University of Vermont in 1895 and practiced in hospitals in Vienna and London.

In Vienna he came into contact with the work of Dr. H. Bressler who had been investigating the possibility of treating organs with pressure points. Through knowledge he gained in Europe and his own research, Fitzgerald found that if pressure was applied on the fingers, it would create a local anesthetic effect on the hand, arm, and shoulder, right up to the jaw, face, ear, and nose. He applied pressure using tight bands of elastic on the middle section of each finger, or by using small clamps that he placed on the tips. He was then able to carry out minor surgical operations using only this pressure technique.[12]

Dr. Fitzgerald divided the body into zones, which he used for his anesthetic effect. By exerting pressure on a specific part of the body he learned to predict which parts of the body would be affected. Fitzgerald established ten equal longitudinal zones running the length of the body from the top of the head to the tips of the toes. The number ten corresponds to the fingers and toes and, therefore,

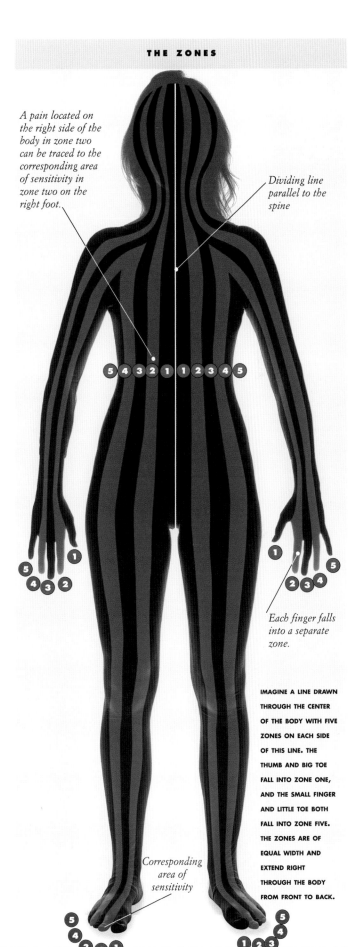

THE ZONES

A pain located on the right side of the body in zone two can be traced to the corresponding area of sensitivity in zone two on the right foot.

Dividing line parallel to the spine

Each finger falls into a separate zone.

Corresponding area of sensitivity

IMAGINE A LINE DRAWN THROUGH THE CENTER OF THE BODY WITH FIVE ZONES ON EACH SIDE OF THIS LINE. THE THUMB AND BIG TOE FALL INTO ZONE ONE, AND THE SMALL FINGER AND LITTLE TOE BOTH FALL INTO ZONE FIVE. THE ZONES ARE OF EQUAL WIDTH AND EXTEND RIGHT THROUGH THE BODY FROM FRONT TO BACK.

11 – ISSEL PP24-5
12 – ANN GILLANDERS "REFLEXOLOGY – THE ANCIENT ANSWER TO MODERN AILMENTS" P35

BELOW
Certain parts of the face deaden sensation in specific areas when pressed.

provides a simple numbering system. Each finger and toe falls into one zone. The theory is that parts of the body found within a certain zone will be linked with one another by the energy flow within the zone and the parts of the body can therefore affect one another.

In his book *Zone Therapy* Fitzgerald describes how he came upon the concept of zone therapy: "I accidentally discovered that pressure with a cotton-tipped probe on the mucocutaneous margin (where the skin joins the mucous membrane) of the nose gave an anaesthetic result as though a cocaine solution had been applied. I further found that there were many spots in the nose, mouth, throat, and on both surfaces of the tongue which, when pressed firmly, deadened definite areas of sensation. Also, that pressures exerted over any body eminence, on the hands, feet, or over the joints, produced the same characteristic result in pain relief. I found also that when pain was relieved, the condition that produced the pain was most generally relieved. This led to my 'mapping out' these various areas and their associated connections, and also noting the conditions influenced through them. This science I have named zone therapy."[13]

PROVING THE THEORY

Fitzgerald and his colleague Dr. Edwin Bowers were so enthusiastic about their discoveries that they developed a unique method for convincing their colleagues about the validity of the zone theory. They would apply pressure to the skeptic's hand then stick a pin in the area of the face anesthetized by the pressure. Such dramatic proof made believers of those who witnessed it. In 1915, Bowers wrote

FAR RIGHT
Zone Therapy, *published in 1917, detailed the work of Doctors Fitzgerald and Bowers but failed to find much support from other physicians.*

the article that first publicly described this treatment and called it "Zone Therapy." This was published in *Everybody's Magazine* and entitled "To Stop that Toothache Squeeze Your Toe!"[14]

PUBLISHED REPORTS

This of course elicited much interest and controversy, and Fitzgerald was often called on to prove publicly the validity of his theories. One such incident was reported in a newspaper on April 29, 1934, under the headline "Mystery of Zone Therapy Explained." The article tells of a dinner party at which one of the guests was Fitzgerald, and another a well-known concert singer who had announced that the upper register tones of her voice had gone flat. Throat specialists had been unable to discover the cause of this affliction. Dr. Fitzgerald asked to examine the fingers and toes of the singer. He told her that the cause of the loss of her upper tones was a callus on her right big toe. After applying pressure to the corresponding part in the same zone for a few minutes, the patient remarked that the pain in her toe had disappeared. Then, to quote from the article: "the doctor asked her to try the tone of the upper register. Miraculously, it would seem to us, the singer reached two tones higher than she had ever done before."[15]

In 1917, the combined work of Dr. Fitzgerald and Dr. Bowers was published in the book *Zone Therapy.* Diagrams of the zones of the feet and the corresponding divisions of the ten zones of the body appeared in the first edition of this book. But the reflex zones of the feet, so crucial to modern reflexology, were not singled out for any special attention by Fitzgerald himself.

Both Fitzgerald and his theories were not enthusiastically received by the medical profession in general, but one

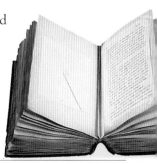

13 – WILLIAM H. FITZGERALD AND EDWIN F. BOWERS "ZONE THERAPY" P9   14 – ISSEL P52
15 – DWIGHT C. BYERS "BETTER HEALTH WITH FOOT REFLEXOLOGY" P3

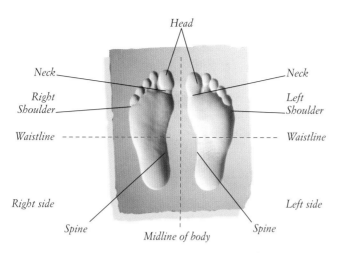

Head

Neck

Right
Shoulder

Waistline

Right side

Spine

Midline of body

Neck

Left
Shoulder

Waistline

Left side

Spine

LEFT
*Eunice Ingham
was the first to
chart a map of the
body on the feet
in 1935.*

physician, Dr. Joseph Shelby Riley, used this method in his practice for many years. Riley refined the techniques and made the first detailed diagrams and drawings of the reflex points located in the feet. He added to Fitzgerald's longitudinal zones his discovery of eight horizontal divisions that also govern the body. His first book *Zone Therapy Simplified* was published in 1919. He wrote four books largely devoted to zone therapy.[16]

EUNICE INGHAM

Fitzgerald, Bowers, and Riley developed and refined the theory of zone therapy, but it was Riley's assistant Eunice Ingham who probably made the greatest contribution to the establishment of modern reflexology. She separated the work on the reflexes of the feet from zone therapy in general.

Eunice Ingham (1879–1974) should be called the Mother of Modern Reflexology. She used zone therapy in her work but felt that the feet should be specific targets for therapy because of their highly sensitive nature. She charted the feet in relation to the zones and their effects on the rest of the anatomy until she had evolved on the feet themselves a "map" of the entire body.

Her nephew Dwight Byers was often a guinea pig for his aunt's research. He recalls: "My earliest recollection of my aunt's work was in 1935 when, during the summer, she lived in Conesus Lake, one of the Finger Lakes in upper New York State. She expanded her research by giving treatments to the residents of this small village. I particularly remember those treatments that year because it was the first time I ever found relief from my annual bouts with asthma and hay fever. She would eagerly practice her theories on my feet while explaining the reflex theory as she worked. I must confess that, to a youth who was wheezing and sneezing, theory took second place to what blessed relief she was able to give me. Interestingly enough, it was while treating me that she convinced herself that in less serious cases, only a few treatments a week sufficed to help most patients."[17]

TEACHING HER THEORIES

Eunice Ingham took her work to the public and the nonmedical community because she realized that lay people could learn the correct reflexology techniques to help themselves, their families, and friends. She was called on to speak at conventions and shared her knowledge with chiropodists, massage practitioners and physiotherapists, naturopaths, and osteopaths. She wrote two books, *Stories The Feet Can Tell* (1938) and *Stories The Feet Have Told* (1963). Today her legacy continues under the direction of her nephew Dwight Byers who runs the International Institute of Reflexology in St. Petersburg.[18]

Zone theory is considered the basis of modern foot reflexology, and most reflexologists use zone therapy as a useful adjunct to their work. However, the time has come to take foot reflexology a step further and expand on existing knowledge by combining it with the ancient Chinese system of meridian therapy.

The Chinese Connection

There can be little doubt that a strong link exists between reflexology and acupuncture. Both techniques are certainly based on similar ideas. Both are considered meridian therapies since they propose that energy lines link the hands and feet to various body parts. This enables the whole body to be treated by working on the reflex areas. Acupuncture went from strength to strength in the East, but reflexology was, for some unknown reason, lost and forgotten until its recent re-emergence in the West.

The Chinese had divided the body into longitudinal meridians by approximately 2500 B.C. whereas the similar idea of zones came to Western awareness as late as the 1900s. Acupuncture, despite its popularity in the East, was an unknown art in the West until 1883 when a Dutch physician, Ten Thyne, wrote a treatise on the subject.

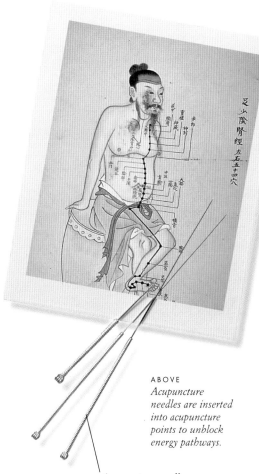

ABOVE
Acupuncture needles are inserted into acupuncture points to unblock energy pathways.

Acupuncture needle

ACUPUNCTURE

Reflexology definitely has some relationship with acupuncture, *shiatsu,* and acupressure. According to acupuncture, the body has 12 pairs of meridians as well as 2 special meridians known as vessels. Together these meridians constitute the body's energy system, which works to maintain the health of the organism. These meridians are pathways through which the energy of the universe circulates throughout the body organs. The flow of life energy also keeps the universe and the body in perfect harmony.

The acupuncturist believes that illness or pain occurs when one or more of the pathways become blocked, disrupting the energy flow and breaking the body's harmony. The Chinese, in acupuncture, developed a technique using needles to unblock these pathways. In *shiatsu,* the Japanese exert direct thumb and finger pressure on these acupuncture meridian points to achieve similar results.[19]

THE MERIDIANS

Reflexologists also work on acupuncture and acupressure points but only those found in the feet. Like the meridians, acupuncture points in the feet mirror those found in other parts of the body. Through increased awareness of meridians one can practice reflexology more effectively as meridians provide profound insight into the disease pathway throughout the body and are therefore a most useful diagnostic tool.

ABOVE
The paths of the meridians through the body, passing through acupuncture meridian points.

19 – ISSEL PP120-21

The Chinese were undoubtedly aware of the importance of the feet in treating disease. In A.D. 1017 Dr. Wang Wei had a human figure cast in bronze on which were marked those points on the body important for acupuncture. When this knowledge was put into practice in treating the sick, practitioners positioned the needles in the appropriate areas of the body and then applied deep pressure therapy on the soles of the inside and outside edge of both feet. They then applied a concentrated pressure on the big toe. The reason they used the feet in conjunction with the acupuncture needles was to channel extra energy through the body. Dr. Wei said that the feet were the most sensitive part of all and contained great energizing areas.[20]

EVIDENCE OF ENERGY PATHWAYS

As more evidence becomes available one can barely refute the fact that, although not visible to the naked eye, energy pathways do exist. Russian physiologists have carried out extensive studies using encephalography, electrocardiography, and X-rays. These studies, which involve measuring the electrical potential of the skin at the classical acupuncture points, have verified basic claims for acupuncture and have also related its effects to reflex action.

To date, most reflexologists have worked with the theory of energy zones originally described by Dr. Fitzgerald. Although his theory has stood reflexology in good stead over the years and contributed greatly to the development of the modern therapy, I personally do not adhere to it. I believe the effects elicited by massaging the feet are largely the result of stimulating the six main meridians that run through the feet. Fitzgerald recognized an energy connection between the feet and other parts of the body, and without his pioneering work reflexology would not be where it is today. But because the Eastern concept of the meridian system was unknown in the West at the time of his research, the connection with the meridians was not recognized. I, however, am convinced that the energy channels linking the feet to other organs and body parts are the meridians described in Chinese medicine.

It is not the object of this book to prove that reflexology is directly related to meridians. The object is to illustrate that a combination of knowledge – modern reflexology techniques and the Eastern meridian system – can be of enormous benefit to both patient and practitioner.

As acupuncture and reflexology are both concerned with balancing energy flow in order to stimulate the body's own healing potential and restore a state of health, and as both therapies are concerned with treating illness and medical conditions in a holistic manner, it seems logical to combine reflexology with meridian therapy in order to provide a more comprehensive and effective treatment program.

LEFT
Small feet were considered the most attractive feature in Chinese women, so their feet were bound from birth to restrict growth, resulting in incredible pain and discomfort. In contrast, ancient Chinese medicine centered on applying pressure techniques to the soles of the feet.

The soles of the feet reflect most of the internal organs
and body systems of the human body. Each foot tells the
patient's case history to the reflexologist.

PART TWO

HOW
REFLEXOLOGY
WORKS

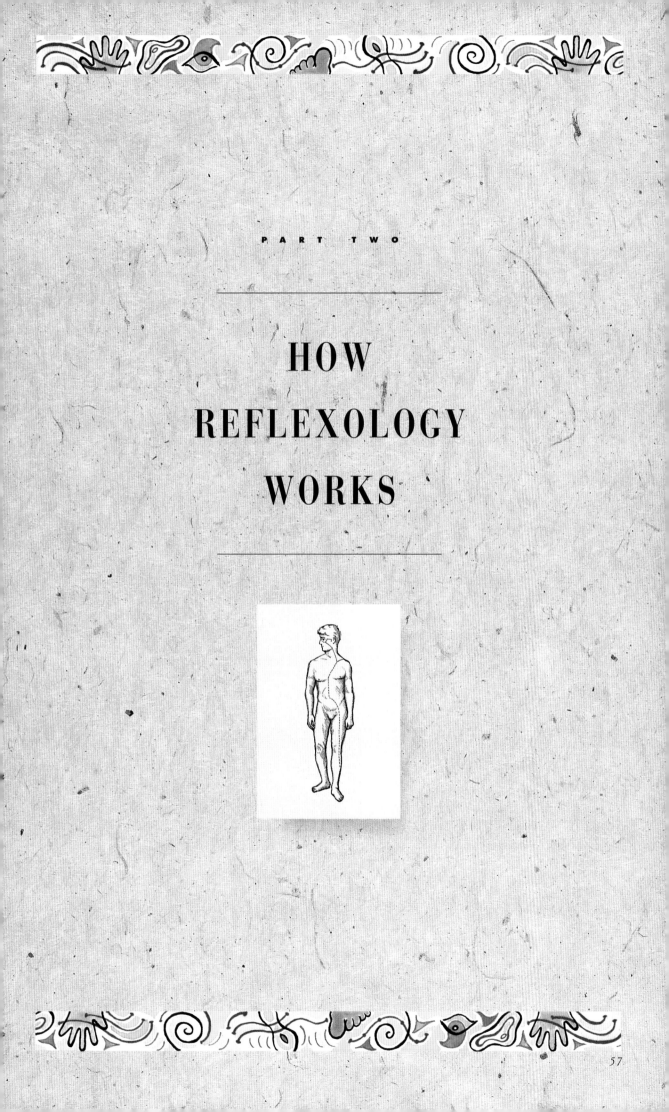

6. THE ANATOMY OF THE FOOT

Few people pay much attention to their feet, which take a severe beating on their path through life. Little notice is given to the serious health damage caused by self-induced foot disorders – disorders that inevitably cause problems elsewhere in the body.

The structure of the foot forms our base and foundation. A strong foundation relies on correct alignments and joint function, and any impairment to the functions will displace the center of gravity. Other areas of the body will then overcompensate causing knee, leg, and calf pain as well as back problems. Poor circulation, incorrect posture, sore backs, and headaches can be attributed to tired, aching feet and swollen ankles. The structure of the foot can be severely damaged by ill-fitting shoes, walking incorrectly, and any other form of excessive stress, such as running and ballet. These conditions cause foot deformities ranging from corns and calluses to more serious damage such as bunions and enlarged toe joints.

Foot deformities and irregularities also affect the reflexes and meridians on which they manifest. This can, in turn, affect the corresponding body parts by causing congestion in energy flow, and possibly affecting associated organs.

To a reflexologist, feet tell a thousand stories. The foot represents the body, and every nick and crevice holds a key to the nature of the problem. A professional, responsible, and successful practitioner will have a thorough knowledge of foot structure meridians and reflexes.

ABOVE, RIGHT, FAR RIGHT
Ballet dancers, followers of fashion, and soccer players make excessive demands on their feet, often suffering from corns, calluses, toenail problems, and muscle and joint strain.

RIGHT
The average foot contains 26 small bones in total; each has a specific job to do.

Calcaneus

Lateral cuneiform

Cuboid bone

Talus

Posterior tubercle of talus

Neck of talus

Head of talus

Navicular

Interm cuneifo

The average foot contains 26 small bones, 2 sesamoids (smaller bones), 114 ligaments, and 20 muscles. These are joined together with connective tissue, blood vessels and nerves and covered with layers of skin. This finely tuned, intricate structure is balanced on two main arches – one, from the heel to the base of the little toe, the other from heel to big toe.

The hands and feet contain the same number of bones – together they make up half the bones of the body. In each foot are 14 phalanges – toe bones. There are three phalanges in each toe, except the big toe, which contains two. These are joined by ligaments to the five metatarsals – long bones that extend the length of the foot toward the heel.

The midfoot is constructed of three cuneiform bones. These help stabilize and support body weight. The longitudinal/transverse arch, which extends from the heel to the ball of the foot, is built of the navicular, cuboid, and the three cuneiform bones.

The heel – calcaneus – bears the brunt of our weight. It is therefore insulated with protective layers of fat to cushion the impact of each footstep. The talus – ankle bone – provides up and down leverage. The joints, muscles, and tendons control the motions of the foot.

It is obvious the foot is a marvelously constructed mechanism. Lamentably, insufficient attention is paid to the feet considering their impressive role in our lives. The common phrase, "My feet are killing me," could be answered with, "You are killing your feet." Reflexology recognizes the vital role of feet in health and healing and aims to emphasize that if you take care of your feet, they will take care of you.

BELOW
This baby's foot is perfectly formed. It is important to make sure shoes fit correctly to try to prevent any deformities in later life.

Flexible, relaxed ankle

Toes do not overlap or rub on shoes.

Well-cushioned heel softens impact of step.

14 Phalanges

Medial cuneiform

5 Metatarsals

7. MERIDIANS: THE VITAL LINK

As we have seen in earlier chapters, the concept of energy channels running through the body is the central point around which the practices of reflexology and acupuncture are founded. In both techniques pressure is applied to specific points to clear blockages of the energy channels.

Meridians and Reflexology

In acupuncture, the lines of vital energy are known as meridians; in reflexology, they are traditionally known as zones. Both ascertain that disease is caused by blockages in energy lines, and treatment involves clearing out these obstructions by stimulating various points along the lines. In acupuncture, points situated all over the body are stimulated by needles. Reflexology concentrates only on reflex areas and sections of meridians found on the feet, which are stimulated by specific massage techniques.

Closer study of the meridians reveals that the six main meridians are found in the feet, specifically the toes. Thus, massaging the feet is, in actual fact, stimulating and clearing congestion in the meridians. When congestions are cleared, energy is able to flow freely and the body is able to achieve a state of balance.

However, since the meridian cycle is one continuous energy flow, the six meridians in the arms that do not penetrate organs are indirectly stimulated when the main meridians are worked on. This is due to the fact that the organs related to these

meridians are found along the six main meridians. For example, the lung meridians run along the arm down to the thumb, but the lung itself is penetrated by the stomach meridian, and therefore congestion would be indirectly affected by stimulating the stomach meridian.

Meridians have a long history. The Chinese discovered the meridian system approximately 3,000 years ago and it has been going from strength to strength. It is a logical progression now to incorporate meridians into the realm of reflexology in order to advance and enhance this holistic health therapy.

An understanding of meridians can help reflexologists to understand the disease pathway more comprehensively, and a basic knowledge of how they work can be of enormous benefit in pinpointing problems. If, for example, pain, irritation, or any other condition does not improve satisfactorily through treatment of the reflex area, one should observe the meridian that traverses the part of the body in question and treat the reflex area of the organ related to that meridian.

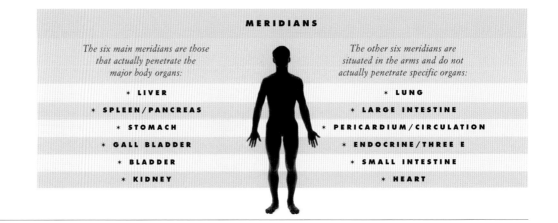

MERIDIANS

The six main meridians are those that actually penetrate the major body organs:

* LIVER
* SPLEEN/PANCREAS
* STOMACH
* GALL BLADDER
* BLADDER
* KIDNEY

The other six meridians are situated in the arms and do not actually penetrate specific organs:

* LUNG
* LARGE INTESTINE
* PERICARDIUM/CIRCULATION
* ENDOCRINE/THREE E
* SMALL INTESTINE
* HEART

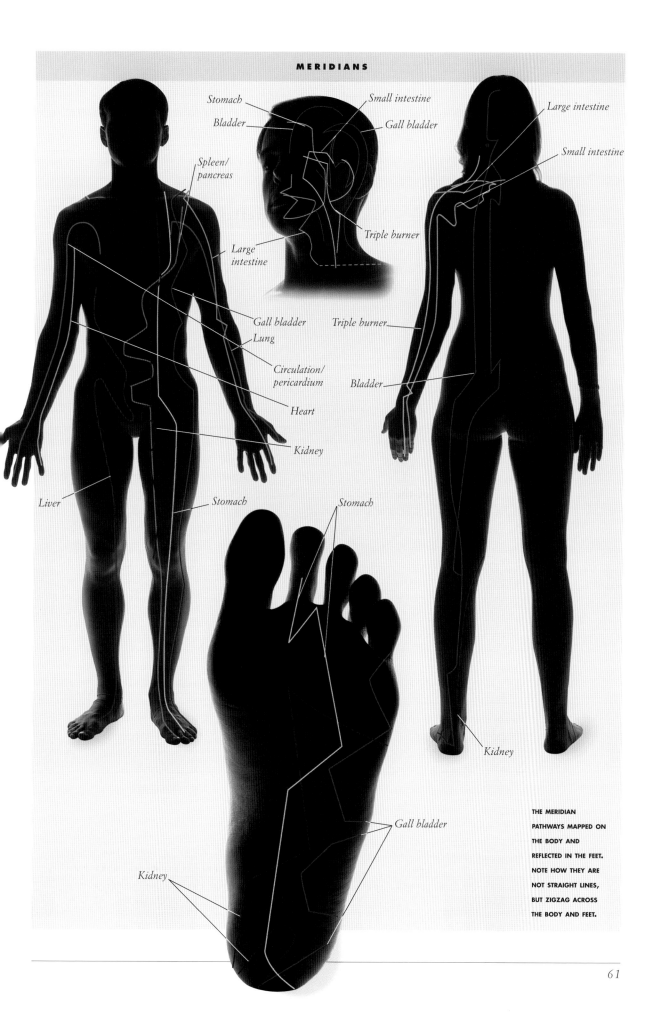

MERIDIANS

Stomach

Bladder

Small intestine

Gall bladder

Large intestine

Small intestine

Spleen/
pancreas

Triple burner

Large
intestine

Gall bladder

Triple burner

Lung

Circulation/
pericardium

Bladder

Heart

Kidney

Liver

Stomach

Stomach

Kidney

Gall bladder

Kidney

THE MERIDIAN
PATHWAYS MAPPED ON
THE BODY AND
REFLECTED IN THE FEET.
NOTE HOW THEY ARE
NOT STRAIGHT LINES,
BUT ZIGZAG ACROSS
THE BODY AND FEET.

What Are Meridians?

We saw in Part 1, page 26 that all life and matter is energy operating at various frequencies. This energy, known as ch'i or life force, is what keeps us alive. The Chinese discovered that this ch'i circulates in the body along "meridians," similar to the blood, nerve, and lymphatic circuits. This vital life force controls the workings of the main organs and systems of the body. It circulates from one organ to another. For each organ to maintain a perfect state of health, the ch'i energy must be able to flow freely along the meridians. If this is balanced, it is impossible to be ill in body, mind, or spirit. All illness is a result of an imbalance in the flow of energy.

Meridians are located throughout the body. They have been described as containing a free-flowing, colorless, noncellular liquid that may be partly actuated by the heart.[1] Meridians have been measured and mapped by modern technological methods, electronically, thermally, and radioactively. With practice they can be felt. There are specific acupuncture points along the meridians. These points are electromagnetic in character and consist of small oval cells called Bonham Corpuscles that surround the capillaries in the skin, the blood vessels, and the organs throughout the body. There are some 500 points that are most frequently used. They are stimulated in a definite sequence depending on the action required. Meridians are named by the live functions with which they seem to associate, so that this name is the same as that of many of the organs we are familiar with.

The Chinese maintain that the ch'i circulates in the meridians 24 times a day and 24 times a night. In a sense, there is

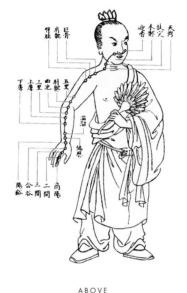

ABOVE

This Chinese illustration shows 40 acu-points along one meridian, counting both sides of the body.

only one single meridian that goes right around the entire body, but many different meridians are described according to their positions and functions. There are 12 main meridians, which are bilateral (paired) resulting in 24 separate pathways. Each meridian is connected and related to a specific organ from which it gets its name. It is also connected to a partner meridian and also an organ with which it has a specific mutual relationship.

Within our bodies the yin organs are those that are hollow and involved in absorption and discharge such as the stomach and the bladder; the yang organs are the dense, blood-filled organs such as the heart, which regulate the body. There is constant interaction between yin and yang forces and, if the yin/yang balance between the organs is interrupted, the

12 MAIN MERIDIANS
* LUNGS
* LARGE INTESTINE
* STOMACH
* SPLEEN/PANCREAS
* HEART
* SMALL INTESTINE
* BLADDER
* KIDNEY
* PERICARDIUM
* "TRIPLE BURNER"
* GALL BLADDER
* LIVER

flow of ch'i throughout the body will be affected and the person will fall ill.

THE MERIDIAN CYCLE

Meridians are classified yin or yang on the basis of the direction in which they flow on the surface of the body. Meridians

1 – JOHN F. THIE "TOUCH FOR HEALTH" P17

interconnect deep within the torso and have an internal branch and a surface branch. The section worked on is the surface branch, which is accessible to touch techniques. Yang energy flows from the sun, and yang meridians run from the fingers to the face, or from the face to the feet. Yin energy from the earth flows from the feet to the torso and from the torso along the inside (yin side) of the arms to the fingertips. Since the meridian flow is actually one long continuous unbroken flow, the energy flows in one definite direction and from one meridian to another in a well-determined order. Because there is no beginning or end to this flow, the order of the meridian is represented as a wheel. As we go around this wheel following the meridian line, the flow moves from torso to fingertips to the face and to the feet before returning to the torso.

The Chinese recognized a 24-hour movement of energy referred to as the Chinese Clock. This "clock" is a 24-hour cycle that divides the day and night into two-hour periods. Each one of these is associated with a surge of energy in one of the organs and its meridian. For example, between the hours of 3 and 5a.m., the lungs receive their daily booster. The cycle begins with the lungs and for this reason it is said that these are the hours when it is most suitable to be born.

The Chinese believe that the best time for stimulating a particular organ is at the two-hour period when its energy is said to be "full." Alternatively, the organ should be sedated at the opposite period of the day or night. For example the lungs should be stimulated between 3 and 5a.m. and sedated between 3 and 5p.m. The opposite treatment should be applied at the opposite time on the clock. The organ maximum energy periods are included in the detailed section on meridians on pages 66–83.

FROM TORSO TO FINGERTIPS, ALONG THE INSIDE OF THE ARM = YIN

FROM FINGERTIPS TO FACE, ALONG THE OUTSIDE/BACK OF THE ARM = YANG

FROM FEET TO TORSO, ALONG THE INSIDE OF THE LEG = YIN

FROM FACE TO FEET, ALONG OUTSIDE OF THE LEG = YANG

LEFT
Energy flows around the body from one meridian to another in a well-defined order. There is no beginning or end to the order – it is best shown as a wheel.

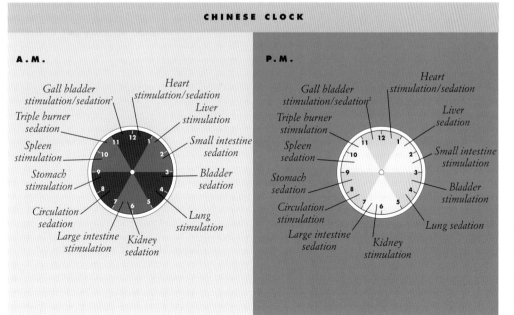

CHINESE CLOCK

A.M.

Gall bladder stimulation/sedation[2]
Triple burner sedation
Spleen stimulation
Stomach stimulation
Circulation sedation
Large intestine stimulation
Kidney sedation
Lung stimulation
Bladder sedation
Small intestine sedation
Liver stimulation
Heart stimulation/sedation

P.M.

Gall bladder stimulation/sedation[2]
Triple burner stimulation
Spleen sedation
Stomach sedation
Circulation stimulation
Large intestine sedation
Kidney stimulation
Lung sedation
Bladder stimulation
Small intestine stimulation
Liver sedation
Heart stimulation/sedation

LEFT
In Chinese medicine, organs are stimulated when their energy is "full" – a specific two-hour period.

2 – THE HEART IS STIMULATED BETWEEN THE HOURS OF 11 A.M. AND 1 P.M. AND SEDATED BETWEEN 11 P.M. AND 1 A.M. AND THE GALL BLADDER IS STIMULATED BETWEEN 11 P.M. AND 1 A.M. AND SEDATED BETWEEN 11 A.M. AND 1 P.M. THESE HAVE, THEREFORE, BEEN INCLUDED ON BOTH A.M. AND P.M. DIAGRAMS.

63

The Five Elements

Each of the five elements is associated with specific parts of the body.

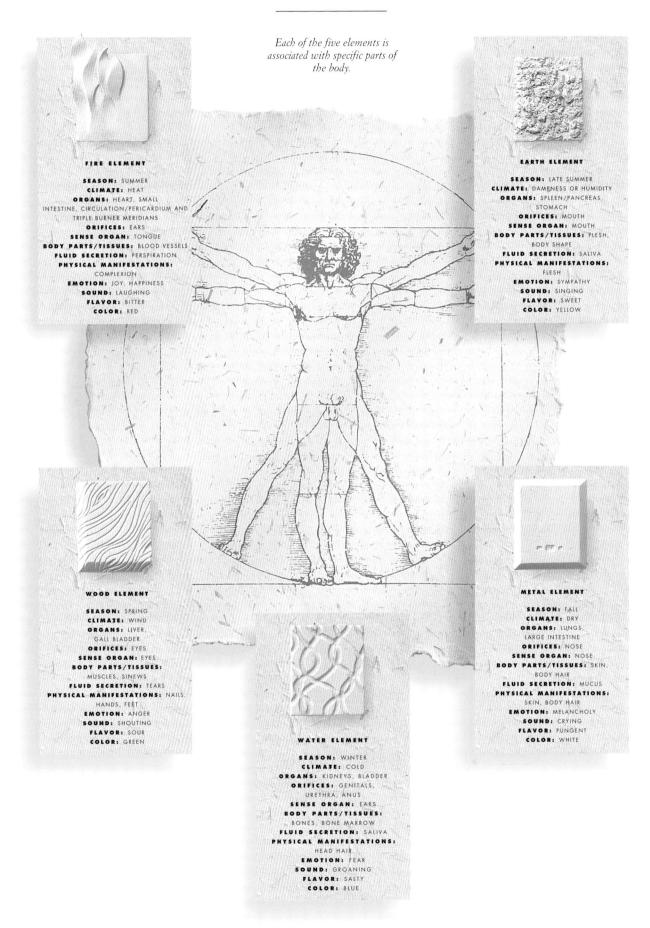

FIRE ELEMENT

SEASON: SUMMER
CLIMATE: HEAT
ORGANS: HEART, SMALL INTESTINE, CIRCULATION/PERICARDIUM AND TRIPLE-BURNER MERIDIANS
ORIFICES: EARS
SENSE ORGAN: TONGUE
BODY PARTS/TISSUES: BLOOD VESSELS
FLUID SECRETION: PERSPIRATION
PHYSICAL MANIFESTATIONS: COMPLEXION
EMOTION: JOY, HAPPINESS
SOUND: LAUGHING
FLAVOR: BITTER
COLOR: RED

EARTH ELEMENT

SEASON: LATE SUMMER
CLIMATE: DAMPNESS OR HUMIDITY
ORGANS: SPLEEN/PANCREAS, STOMACH
ORIFICES: MOUTH
SENSE ORGAN: MOUTH
BODY PARTS/TISSUES: FLESH, BODY SHAPE
FLUID SECRETION: SALIVA
PHYSICAL MANIFESTATIONS: FLESH
EMOTION: SYMPATHY
SOUND: SINGING
FLAVOR: SWEET
COLOR: YELLOW

WOOD ELEMENT

SEASON: SPRING
CLIMATE: WIND
ORGANS: LIVER, GALL BLADDER
ORIFICES: EYES
SENSE ORGAN: EYES
BODY PARTS/TISSUES: MUSCLES, SINEWS
FLUID SECRETION: TEARS
PHYSICAL MANIFESTATIONS: NAILS, HANDS, FEET
EMOTION: ANGER
SOUND: SHOUTING
FLAVOR: SOUR
COLOR: GREEN

METAL ELEMENT

SEASON: FALL
CLIMATE: DRY
ORGANS: LUNGS, LARGE INTESTINE
ORIFICES: NOSE
SENSE ORGAN: NOSE
BODY PARTS/TISSUES: SKIN, BODY HAIR
FLUID SECRETION: MUCUS
PHYSICAL MANIFESTATIONS: SKIN, BODY HAIR
EMOTION: MELANCHOLY
SOUND: CRYING
FLAVOR: PUNGENT
COLOR: WHITE

WATER ELEMENT

SEASON: WINTER
CLIMATE: COLD
ORGANS: KIDNEYS, BLADDER
ORIFICES: GENITALS, URETHRA, ANUS
SENSE ORGAN: EARS
BODY PARTS/TISSUES: BONES, BONE MARROW
FLUID SECRETION: SALIVA
PHYSICAL MANIFESTATIONS: HEAD HAIR
EMOTION: FEAR
SOUND: GROANING
FLAVOR: SALTY
COLOR: BLUE

Meridian therapy and acupuncture can be understood more clearly in the light of the Chinese belief that five elements comprise the world, and that everything on earth essentially falls into the category of one or more of these elements. These elements are wood, fire, earth, metal, and water. The five elements do not refer to material elements, but rather conditions, or states.

The five elements are generated and destroyed according to a law of cyclical interaction: fire produces earth, earth produces metal, metal finds water, water produces wood, and wood becomes fire. By substituting for each element a corresponding yin organ, for example, we see that the heart (fire) aids or reinforces the action of the spleen/pancreas (earth); the spleen/pancreas the lungs (metal); the lungs the kidneys (water); the kidneys the liver (wood); and the liver the heart.

Although the stomach is referred to as an earth organ, and the kidneys a water organ, remember that these inner organs are classified according to element dominance. All organs have traces of the four others, and it is through these traces that an organ is linked with other organs of a different element and the element's "pool." For example, the metal organs, lungs and large intestine, are linked through their water element trace with the water organs, kidneys and bladder; or through their wood element trace with the wood organs, liver and gall bladder.[3]

Each of these elements is associated with a variety of factors: for example, body organs, sense organs, body tissue, colors, emotions, seasons, climate, and more. Any extreme reactions to any of these factors (for example, either a strong aversion to or an increased desire for any specific color, season, or taste) can indicate an imbalance in a related element. That element can then in turn be related to the organs and meridians of the body (see pages 68–83), and, in this way, can be used as an additional diagnostic tool.

A person who seems wellrooted and has a flexible approach to life will be strong in the wood element, whose season is spring – a time of generation of new life and the ability to be creative, and capable of change. If such a person is disturbed, that person could become off-balance, uprooted, and easily confused.

Emotions are also important in the diagnostic process. The fire element relates to love, happiness, gentleness, and forgiveness. The element stimulates both physical body warmth, and psychological warmth in our relationships with others. Lack of concern and love for others, as well as lack of energy to love oneself, is indicative of an imbalance on the emotional plane.

If we look at taste, we find that each flavor has an effect on energy. The combination of five tastes ensures balance. An excess of one flavor can have an injurious effect, yet each element can be strengthened if the right flavor is prescribed for it.[4] The same applies to color. Color can also be perceived in the face. If ch'i is flowing harmoniously, the face will not show any predominant color, but if one element is imbalanced the color associated with it will show as a subtle hue.

Other element correspondences relating to the body functions are closely related to organ function. Any disturbances related to these organs also clearly indicate specific energy imbalances within a particular element.

ELEMENT	YIN/YANG	ORGAN
FIRE	YIN	HEART, PERICARDIUM/ CIRCULATION
	YANG	SMALL INTESTINE TRIPLE BURNER
EARTH	YIN	SPLEEN/PANCREAS
	YANG	STOMACH
METAL	YIN	LUNGS
	YANG	LARGE INTESTINE
WATER	YIN	KIDNEYS
	YANG	BLADDER
WOOD	YIN	LIVER
	YANG	GALL BLADDER

ABOVE
Each of the five elements is affected by both of the dynamic complementary forces – yin and yang. The organs are governed by one of these two forces.

3 – D. & J. LAWSON-WOOD "FIVE ELEMENTS OF ACUPUNCTURE & CHINESE MASSAGE" P40
4 – DIANNE M. CONNELLY, PH.D. MAC. "TRADITIONAL ACUPUNCTURE: THE LAW OF THE FIVE ELEMENTS" P25

The Meridians in Detail

Kidney meridian

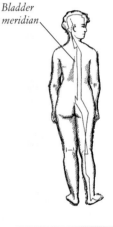

ABOVE
The kidney meridian affects the throat (internal branch), lungs, heart, breast, solar plexus, diaphragm, groin, leg, uterus/prostate, and bladder.

The meridians can be used simply and effectively for a better understanding of a wide range of conditions affecting the body.

A disorder in the stom-ach meridian, for example, may cause upper toothache because the meridian passes through the upper gums. Lower toothache may be the result of a disorder of the large intestine meridian. Pain in the groin may as easily result from a liver meridian disorder as from a disorder of the liver itself.

Another example could be a person with arthritis in the little finger, tennis elbow, fibrositis in the shoulder blade, infection of the lymph glands in the throat, trigeminal neuralgia, and hearing problems. One need simply look at the small intestine meridian – this starts in the little finger, ends just in front of the ear, and passes the locations of all of the above disorders. Could this mean that a small intestine disorder could aggravate or even cause these problems? Clinical results of balancing the meridians indicate that it could do so.

Stomach meridian

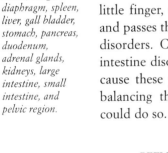

ABOVE
The stomach meridian (its internal branch represented by a dotted line) affects the sinuses, throat, lungs, diaphragm, spleen, liver, gall bladder, stomach, pancreas, duodenum, adrenal glands, kidneys, large intestine, small intestine, and pelvic region.

BELOW
The spleen/pancreas meridian affects the throat and thyroid (internal branch), underarm, digestion, pelvis, thigh, knee, and skin.

REFLEXOLOGY "DIAGNOSIS"

In most countries reflexologists are not allowed to diagnose any specific conditions. In my work as a teacher and practitioner I have found it important that a client understands the nature of his or her complaints and so will be more willing to cooperate with any advice. In order to understand the complaint, the practitioner requires a detailed case history of all symptoms, not only those that are the cause of the most severe problems

Spleen/ pancreas meridian

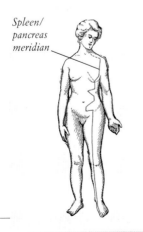

at the time of consultation. The complaints can then be related to the meridians in order to ascertain which of the organs are out of balance. Instead of using the symptoms to diagnose a medical condition, one must understand them in accordance with the Chinese philosophy of blockage in energy flow.

COMPLETE TREATMENT

Study of the path of the 12 meridians shows that the stomach meridian penetrates all the major organs in the body as well as passing through all the reflexes of the major organs in the feet. This is the dominant meridian, often the root cause of congestion.

It is important to do a complete treatment in each case, no matter what the symptoms, rather than to work only on those reflexes one may believe to be congested. Weakness may be expressed in congestions of ch'i energy at any point along the meridian, not just in the actual organs.

The case histories in this section have all been effectively treated with the techniques described in this book, which clear congestions, allowing both the energy to flow freely and the body to reach a state of balance. We will now examine individual meridians in depth and look at the sort of illnesses and conditions each is associated with.

Bladder meridian

ABOVE
The bladder meridian affects the central nervou. system of the spinal cord, nerves and brain indirectly affecting all the body's organs.

PATIENT HISTORY

Severe back pain leading to pain down the legs. Has had a fusion of lumbar vertebrae 3 and 4 a few years ago. Has had more pain since then. Suffering from depression and despair (Wood Element). Breathing is very shallow.

When she walks a lot she needs to urinate more and the urine burns (this condition has occurred since the fusion in her vertebrae (above), since lumbar vertebrae 3 is connected to the bladder).

Teeth are dry (Water Element).

Often has pain in her right kidney.

Suffers from a lot of phobias.

Energy level is low in the afternoons (Water Element).

Hysterectomy six years ago because her uterus was full of fibroids. At the same time she had a bladder repair.

Other operations: tonsils, lump in right breast.

Bowel movement is 1-2 times a week on laxatives – feels bloated and windy.

Skin on her face is dry (Metal Element).

Thumbs and index fingers are often "sore."

Strong desire for coffee and sweet food (Earth Element).

Diet: Very acid, consisting of toast with cheese for breakfast. Protein (red meat) with bread for lunch, and fruits and bread for supper. Drinks lots of water in the belief that she needs to "flush" out her system.

Hardly any vegetables.

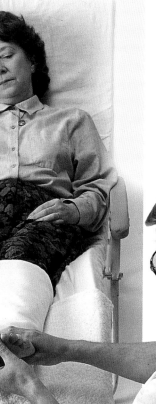

LEFT
At the start of a reflexology treatment the practitioner takes a detailed case history and discusses the complaint and its treatment with the client.

LUNG MERIDIAN

YIN MERIDIAN	PARTNER MERIDIAN: LARGE INTESTINE - YANG
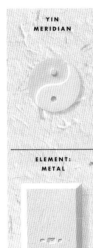	
ELEMENT: METAL	ORGAN MAXIMUM ENERGY PERIOD: 3A.M. TO 5A.M.

The lungs and large intestine control elimination: the former carbon dioxide, the latter solid residue. Since these meridians are partnered, they can directly affect each other – for example, chest problems can be accompanied by constipation, and constipation can be accompanied by chest problems.

The lungs regulate respiration. They are responsible for taking ch'i from the air and for regulating the states of ch'i in the body. Healthy lungs and regular, even respiration ensure that ch'i enters and leaves the body smoothly. An imbalance results in symptoms such as asthma, coughs, and various forms of chest congestion. Respiratory functions affect all the rhythms of the body, including the blood flow.

The lungs are called the "tender" organ because they are the most easily influenced by environmental factors and are involved with regulating sweat secretions, which increase resistance to external environmental influences.

Shoulder pain, supraclavicular fossa

Stiff forearm

Skin problems

Wrist disorders, carpal tunnel syndrome

Arthritis or stiffness in the thumb, warts

White spots on thumbnail, ridges on nail, whitlow

THE LUNG MERIDIAN STARTS AT THE CLAVICLE AND ENDS AT THE BACK OF THE THUMB TOWARD THE INDEX FINGER.

LARGE INTESTINE MERIDIAN

The large intestine forms the lower part of the digestive tract and is in charge of transporting, transforming, and eliminating surplus matter. If these wastes are not eliminated regularly, it can have a toxic effect on the entire system. Thus mental constipation – toxic thoughts and feelings – are often associated with this meridian, in addition to physical constipation or diarrhea.[6]

The *Nei Ching* refers to the large intestine as the generator of evolution and change – and as being integral to the well-being of the whole body. The important function of elimination of waste material is vital to the maintenance of health. If waste is not effectively excreted, the rest of the system has to cope with an additional load of toxic waste and this will cause disharmony throughout the body. An imbalance in the large intestine can result in abdominal pain, diarrhea, constipation, bloatedness, swelling, acne and boils, headaches, and stuffy nose.

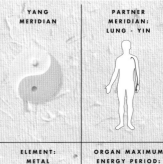

YANG MERIDIAN

PARTNER MERIDIAN: LUNG - YIN

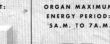

ELEMENT: METAL

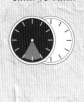

ORGAN MAXIMUM ENERGY PERIOD: 5A.M. TO 7A.M.

Bleeding nose, sores in the nose

Herpes/cold sores on the lips

Shoulder pain, frozen shoulder, bursitis

Skin problems

Tennis elbow

Arthritis in the index fingers, eczema, white spots on fingernails, ridges on nail, whitlow

THE LARGE INTESTINE (COLON) MERIDIAN STARTS FROM THE TIP OF THE INDEX FINGER, CROSSES THE BACK OF THE SHOULDER AND ENDS ON THE FACE AT EITHER SIDE OF THE NOSE.

STOMACH MERIDIAN

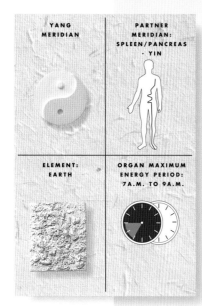

YANG MERIDIAN	PARTNER MERIDIAN: SPLEEN/PANCREAS - YIN
ELEMENT: EARTH	ORGAN MAXIMUM ENERGY PERIOD: 7A.M. TO 9A.M.

The functions and activities of the stomach and spleen are closely related. The stomach controls digestion – it receives nourishment, integrates it and passes on the "pure" food energy to be distributed by the spleen. The spleen then transforms it into the raw material for ch'i and blood. If the stomach does not hold and digest food, the spleen cannot transform it and transmit its essence. The stomach and spleen are interdependent meridians.

According to Chinese philosophy, the stomach is related to appetite, digestion, and transportation of food and liquid, but the ruler of food transportation and energy consumption is the stomach's partner, the spleen/pancreas.

Lung/bronch problems

Blemishes

Eye weakness, goiter

Sinus pain

Checks (capillaries)

Skin marks, acne, birthmarks

Tonsilitis, sore throat, laryngitis, thyroid problems

Breast (nipple) soreness, sore breast, lumps, inverted nipples

Diaphragm disorders, e.g. hiatus hernia; liver/gall bladder disorders (right side); stomach, pancreas, and spleen disorders (left side)

Kidney/adrenal disorders, allergies

Digestive problems, e.g. constipation, diverticulitis, colic, hernia

Appendix (right side) and ovarian problems, blocked Fallopian tubes, infertility

Thigh pain

Knee pain, eczema, psoriasis, shinbone problems, varicose veins

Corns, fungus on the nail, hammer toe, malformed toe

THE STOMACH MERIDIAN STARTS UNDER THE EYE AND CURVES UP TO THE TEMPLE AND THEN CONTINUES DOWN THE BODY AND ENDS ON THE TOP OF THE SECOND TOE.

ABERDEEN
236 Union Street
Aberdeen AB1 1TN
Telephone 01224 571655
Facsimile 01224 213667

DUNDEE
35 Commercial Street
Dundee DD1 3DG
Telephone 01382 200322
Facsimile 01382 201730

EDINBURGH
128 Princes Street
Edinburgh EH2 4AD
Telephone 0131 226 2666
Facsimile 0131 226 4689

13 Princes Street
Edinburgh EH2 2AN
Telephone 0131 556 3034/5
Facsimile 0131 557 8801

83 George Street
Edinburgh EH2 3ES
Telephone 0131 225 3436
Facsimile 0131 226 4548

GLASGOW
132 Union Street
Glasgow G1 3QH
Telephone 0141 221 0890
Facsimile 0141 221 4067

45 Princes Square
Glasgow G1 3JN
Telephone 0141 221 9650

PERTH
St. John's Centre
Perth
Scotland PH1 5UX
Telephone 01738 630013
Facsimile 01738 643478

MAILING SERVICE
Telephone 01225 448595
Facsimile 01225 444732
Facsimile 01225 420575

Books to catch
the moment
t Waterstone's

rth element work together more
stabilize the individual. The earth
d if there is no harmony in the
this will affect all the other

y the Chinese as the "sea of
s digestion and is responsi-
ng" ingested foods and flu-
ctivities of the stomach the
d not function. The stomach
tionally; thus, according to
m occurring in the stomach is
organs.
ce, whatever is taken in, be it
ill not be utilized correctly.
gy,

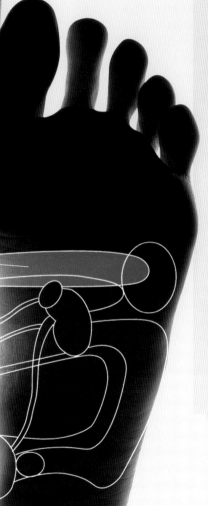

**THE STOMACH REFLEX IS FOUND
ON THE SOLES OF BOTH FEET.**

CASE STUDY

FEMALE: AGE – 35

SYMPTOMS
Chronic sinusitis, PMS, and menstrual
pains; used a contraceptive pill for
pain relief and to suppress facial acne;
radical mood swings; fatigue, heartburn, and constipation.

PREVIOUS OPERATIONS
Part of an overactive thyroid removed;
she now takes a prescription drug for
this condition.

REFLEXOLOGY
To help her body cope without the aid
of the contraceptive pill. Made aware
of the pathway of the stomach meridian and the need to modify diet to
exclude acidic foods and increase
alkaline foods. First period off the pill
was heavy, but the PMS had lessened.
The heartburn decreased. After three
treatments, constipation was no
longer a problem. Had suffered only
one bad sinus attack and the acne
was insignificant. Had second menstrual cycle after the fifth reflexology
treatment and suffered no pain, only
slight PMS and the cycle was lighter
and also shorter.

SPLEEN/PANCREAS MERIDIAN

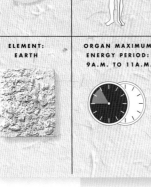

YIN MERIDIAN	PARTNER MERIDIAN: STOMACH - YANG
ELEMENT: EARTH	ORGAN MAXIMUM ENERGY PERIOD: 9A.M. TO 11A.M.

A traditional saying that combines the meaning of several references in the *Nei Ching* states that "the spleen rules transformation and transportation."[7] It is the crucial link in the process by which food is transformed into ch'i and blood. If this process of food transformation is not activated, nourishment and ch'i are not available for the muscles so they become weak and the lips and mouth become pale and dry. The spleen is traditionally referred to as the "foundation of postnatal existence." If the spleen is imbalanced the whole body or some part of it may develop deficient ch'i or deficient blood.

Problems with outer breast (sore, lumps, etc.)

Underarm complaints (e.g. eczema, boils, and lymph swellings)

Abdominal pain

Pelvic complaints e.g. cysts, fibroids in the uterus

Menstrual problems, infections

Groin pain, hernias

Thigh pain, varicose veins, psoriasis

Knee pain (inner side)

Shinbone problems, eczema

Fungus, stiffness, or ingrowing toenails

Outer edge of big toe relates to the spleen/pancreas meridian

THE SPLEEN/PANCREAS MERIDIAN STARTS AT THE TIP OF THE BIG TOE, RUNS UP THE LEG, BENDS INTO THE PELVIS, RUNS UP THE SIDE OF THE ABDOMEN, AND ENDS AT THE SHOULDER.

Bunions

7 – THE "HUANG-DI NEI-CHING" OR THE "YELLOW EMPEROR'S CLASSIC OF INTERNAL MEDICINE" REFERRED TO AS THE BIBLE OF CHINESE MEDICINE AND DATING BACK ABOUT 4,500 YEARS. ILZA VEITH "THE YELLOW EMPEROR'S CLASSIC OF INTERNAL MEDICINE" P133.

Physiologically, the pancreas has considerable control over the body's nourishment, since its secretions help digest all the main kinds of food: proteins, fats, and starch.

According to the Chinese, "The spleen governs the blood"; it helps create blood and keeps it flowing in its correct paths. It therefore also influences menstruation. The spleen destroys spent red blood cells and forms antibodies that neutralize poisonous bacteria, thus influencing immunity to infection. Another important function of this meridian has to do with the transformation of liquids; the classics say that edema (swelling from retention of excess fluids) is related to the spleen.

Pancreas reflex

Spleen reflex

CASE STUDY

FEMALE: AGE – 40

SYMPTOMS
Daily headaches; constipation; sweet tooth; regular menstrual cycle but heavy with slight cramps.

PREVIOUS OPERATIONS
Bunion removed: lumpectomy performed on right breast.

REFLEXOLOGY
Daily headaches which indicate an imbalance on the bladder meridian. This case was more of a problem with the spleen/pancreas and its meridian, since the other symptoms and operations noted were largely on the spleen/pancreas meridian. The effect of the imbalance was manifested in the form of headaches.

THE PANCREAS REFLEXES ARE FOUND ON THE SOLES OF BOTH FEET. THE SPLEEN REFLEX IS FOUND ON THE SOLE OF THE LEFT FOOT.

SMALL INTESTINE MERIDIAN

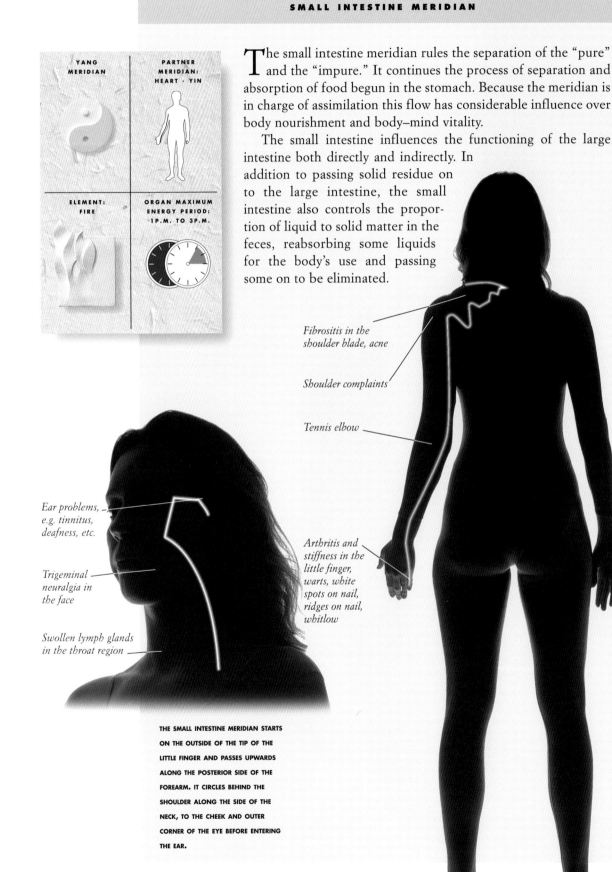

YANG
MERIDIAN

PARTNER
MERIDIAN:
HEART - YIN

ELEMENT:
FIRE

ORGAN MAXIMUM
ENERGY PERIOD:
1P.M. TO 3P.M.

The small intestine meridian rules the separation of the "pure" and the "impure." It continues the process of separation and absorption of food begun in the stomach. Because the meridian is in charge of assimilation this flow has considerable influence over body nourishment and body–mind vitality.

The small intestine influences the functioning of the large intestine both directly and indirectly. In addition to passing solid residue on to the large intestine, the small intestine also controls the proportion of liquid to solid matter in the feces, reabsorbing some liquids for the body's use and passing some on to be eliminated.

Fibrositis in the
shoulder blade, acne

Shoulder complaints

Tennis elbow

Ear problems,
e.g. tinnitus,
deafness, etc.

Arthritis and
stiffness in the
little finger,
warts, white
spots on nail,
ridges on nail,
whitlow

Trigeminal
neuralgia in
the face

Swollen lymph glands
in the throat region

THE SMALL INTESTINE MERIDIAN STARTS
ON THE OUTSIDE OF THE TIP OF THE
LITTLE FINGER AND PASSES UPWARDS
ALONG THE POSTERIOR SIDE OF THE
FOREARM. IT CIRCLES BEHIND THE
SHOULDER ALONG THE SIDE OF THE
NECK, TO THE CHEEK AND OUTER
CORNER OF THE EYE BEFORE ENTERING
THE EAR.

The "sorting out" process – keeping that which has value and passing on waste to where it can be removed – happens on all levels, both physiological and psychological, for example in sorting out the "rubbish" from that which is useful in terms of ideas, emotions, and thoughts. If this function is not operating efficiently symptoms that express this confusion may arise – for example hearing difficulties, such as the inability to distinguish different sounds. Thus the flow relates not only to assimilation of foodstuffs but also to assimilation of experience, feelings, and ideas and to spiritual nourishment.

CASE STUDY

FEMALE: AGE – EARLY 30s

SYMPTOMS

Severe neck, back, and shoulder problem – pinched sensation from shoulder down the arm and at one point she lost all feelings in her arm; weak stomach – often experiences cramps after meals; weakness in throat; tennis elbow; at the age of six had a hernia in the groin; at age five suffered a severe ear infection that caused balance problems.

REFLEXOLOGY

Problems along the small intestine meridian were obvious in the symptoms of the shoulder, neck/arm, elbow, ear, and throat. Meridians in the arms do not penetrate any major organs and one would have to look for the cause on one of the main meridians and the related organs. The weak stomach and cramps after meals indicate a stomach imbalance. But the ch'i energy congestions are located mainly along the arm, shoulder, neck, ears, and throat.

Small intestine reflex

THE SMALL INTESTINE REFLEX IS FOUND
ON THE SOLES OF BOTH FEET.

HEART MERIDIAN

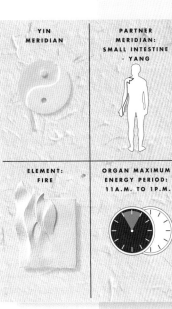

YIN MERIDIAN	PARTNER MERIDIAN: SMALL INTESTINE - YANG
ELEMENT: FIRE	ORGAN MAXIMUM ENERGY PERIOD: 11A.M. TO 1P.M.

The heart and small intestine meridians are coupled; the *Nei Ching* explains their relationship: "The heart controls the blood and unites with the small intestine. If the heart becomes heated, the heat will converge in the small intestine, producing blood in the urine."[8]

The classics say, "The heart rules the blood and blood vessels." It regulates the blood flow, so when the heart is functioning correctly, the blood flows smoothly. If the heart is strong, the body will be healthy and the emotions orderly; if it is weak, all the other meridians will be disturbed in consequence.

It is also said that the heart rules the spirit. So, when the heart's blood and ch'i are harmonious, spirit is nourished and the individual responds appropriately to the environment. If this is impaired symptoms such as insomnia, excessive dreaming, forgetfulness, hysteria, irrational behavior, insanity, and delirium may manifest.

Pain in the armpits, swollen glands

Inner arm pain and weakness, numbness, angina

Weak wrists

Stiffness or pain in the little finger, ridges on nail, white spots on nail, warts, whitlow

THE HEART MERIDIAN STARTS IN THE ARMPIT AND ENDS AT THE BACK OF THE LITTLE FINGER TOWARD THE RING FINGER.

8 – IONA MARSAA-TEEGURDEN "HANDBOOK OF ACUPRESSURE" P12

BLADDER MERIDIAN

The partnership of the kidneys and bladder meridians is one of the most obvious and means that the bladder meridian has a role in stimulating and regulating the kidneys.

The function of the bladder is to receive and excrete urine produced in the kidneys, and the meridian is, therefore, in charge of maintaining normal fluid levels in the body. It is also coupled with the function of the kidney in helping to store the vital essence (see "Kidney Meridian"). The bladder is essential to life because if it is not functioning, the rest of the system becomes poisoned and stressed beyond endurance.

The bladder meridian strongly affects the spinal cord and nerves and it is most effective in releasing tensions along its route.

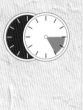

YANG MERIDIAN	PARTNER MERIDIAN: KIDNEY - YIN
ELEMENT: WATER	ORGAN MAXIMUM ENERGY PERIOD: 3 P.M. TO 5 P.M.

Headaches (including forehead and sinus), eye weaknesses (red or weak eyes)

Pain and stiffness along spine

Weak, sore lower back

Hemorrhoids, boils on the buttocks

Hair loss

Neck tension

Sciatica, varicose veins

Tightness and pain in calf, cramps

Weak feet, weak ankles, athlete's foot, bent little toes, or pigeon toes

THE BLADDER MERIDIAN STARTS AT THE INNER CORNER OF THE EYE, CONTINUES OVER THE CROWN OF THE HEAD, DOWN THE BACK OF THE LEGS AND ENDS ON THE OUTER EDGE OF THE BACK OF THE LITTLE TOE.

KIDNEY MERIDIAN

YIN MERIDIAN	PARTNER MERIDIAN: BLADDER – YANG
ELEMENT: WATER	ORGAN MAXIMUM ENERGY PERIOD: 5 P.M. TO 7 P.M.

The *Nei Ching* states: "When the kidneys are deficient . . . the spirit becomes easily provoked."[9]

The kidneys store the jing and rule birth, development, and maturation. Jing is the substance – a vital essence – that is the source of life and individual development. It has the potential for differentiation to yin and yang and, therefore, produces life. The body and all the organs need jing to thrive, and because the kidneys store jing, they bestow this potential for life activity. They have a special relationship with the other organs because the yin

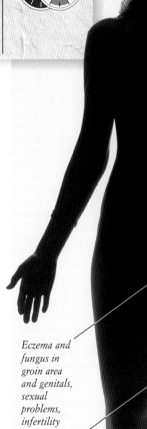

Lung congestion

Breast lumps (on the inner side of the nipple)

Heart

Solar plexus and diaphragm problems

Bladder weakness

Phlebitis on inner calves

Shinbone sores (inner side)

Swollen inner ankles

Eczema and fungus in groin area and genitals, sexual problems, infertility

Thigh pain, varicose veins

Burning, painful soles of the feet, eczema, and fungus on the soles

THE KIDNEY MERIDIAN STARTS ON THE SOLE OF THE FOOT AND ASCENDS UP THE BACK OF THE LEG. IT EMERGES AROUND THE FRONT OF THE LOWER THIGH AND ASCENDS STRAIGHT UP THE BODY TO THE BREASTBONE.

9 – VEITH
P133

and yang, or life activity of each organ, ultimately depends on the ying and yang of the kidneys.

The kidneys regulate the amount of water in the body. Fluid is essential to life. The flow of the fluid enables waste material to be collected and excreted in the form of urine. Enormous amounts of blood flow through the kidneys to be purified. If the blood does not flow as it should symptoms such as high blood pressure or hypertension may result and there may be a buildup of toxic substances that the body would be unable to deal with.

CASE STUDY

MALE: AGE – MID-60s

SYMPTOMS

General bad circulation; painful calves; tingling burning sensation on the feet; has to get up every night in order to urinate.

PREVIOUS OPERATIONS

Three bypass operations; lumpectomy on the elbow.

REFLEXOLOGY

Reference to the kidney meridian shows that the heart is situated on its pathway. The burning area on the feet was around the kidney reflexes found there. Five plantar warts were situated on the heart reflex of the foot. The lump on the elbow can be traced to the heart meridian. Problems with the calf muscle relate to the partner meridian, the bladder.

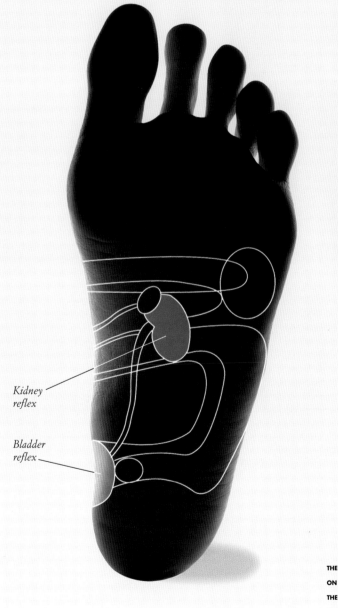

Kidney reflex

Bladder reflex

THE KIDNEY REFLEXES ARE FOUND ON THE SOLES OF BOTH FEET AND THE BLADDER ON THE INSIDE PART OF BOTH FEET.

CIRCULATION/PERICARDIUM MERIDIAN

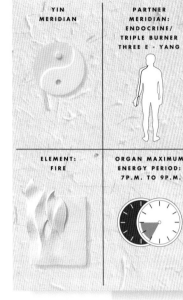

YIN MERIDIAN	PARTNER MERIDIAN: ENDOCRINE/ TRIPLE BURNER THREE E - YANG
ELEMENT: FIRE	ORGAN MAXIMUM ENERGY PERIOD: 7 P.M. TO 9 P.M.

The pericardium and triple burner are coupled meridians and both have protective functions. The pericardium protects the heart – the ruler – and the triple burner protects the other nine meridians. The condition of either affects the other; if the triple burner is imbalanced, the organs are deprived of proper nourishment and revolt against the heart; if the pericardium is weak, the heart will be attacked and the nourishing activities of the triple burner will be less effective.

One main function of the meridian is to protect the heart – physically as well as energetically. The pericardium is a fibrous sac enclosing a slippery lubricated membrane that prevents friction as the heart beats. Stresses and shocks first affect the pericardium and do not penetrate the heart unless the pericardium is weakened.

Swollen, painful armpits (axilla swollen)

Eczema or skin problems in the elbow crease

Hot palms

Carpal tunnel syndrome

Arthritis/eczema in the middle finger, warts, whitlow, white spots on nail, ridges on nail

THE CIRCULATION/PERICARDIUM MERIDIAN HAS A DESCENDING FLOW RUNNING FROM THE CHEST TO THE HAND. IT STARTS NEXT TO THE NIPPLE AND DESCENDS DOWN THE ARM ENDING ON THE BACK OF THE MIDDLE FINGER TOWARD THE RING FINGER.

TRIPLE BURNER/ENDOCRINE/THREE E MERIDIAN

The triple burner meridian is the partner of the circulation meridian. Though there is no anatomical organ that correlates with the triple burner, the Chinese believe that all the organs in the body are guarded by it and that heat in the body is controlled by this function.

The three "heaters" or "burners" correspond to divisions of the torso: the upper burner to the thoracic cavity; the middle burner to the abdominal cavity; the lower burner to the pelvic cavity. Their functions include:

• regulation of the autonomic nervous system and thus of the heart and abdominal organs especially in their response to emotion
• control of the pituitary gland
• regulation of body temperature, appetite, and thirst
• control of emotions and moods – the urges of pleasure and displeasure.

Shoulder pains

Pain behind and in the outer corner of the eye

Ear problems e.g. pain, eczema, and gout

Arthritis, white spots or ridges on the nail of third finger, eczema on the fourth finger, warts, whitlow

Stiffness and pain along the arm and wrist

YANG MERIDIAN

PARTNER MERIDIAN: PERICARDIUM - YIN

ELEMENT: FIRE

ORGAN MAXIMUM ENERGY PERIOD: 9P.M. TO 11P.M.

THE TRIPLE BURNER MERIDIAN STARTS ON THE BACK OF THE RING FINGER, ASCENDS UP THE ARM AND ENDS AT THE TOP OF THE OUTER CORNER OF THE EYE.

GALL BLADDER MERIDIAN

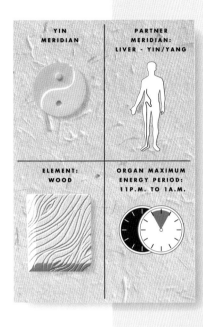

YIN MERIDIAN

PARTNER MERIDIAN: LIVER - YIN/YANG

ELEMENT: WOOD

ORGAN MAXIMUM ENERGY PERIOD: 11P.M. TO 1A.M.

It is essential to note that the Chinese think of the organs as functions operating on all levels of the body–mind . . . "the liver has the functions of a military leader who excels in his strategic planning; the gall bladder occupies the position of an important and upright official who excels through his decisions and judgement."[10]

According to the Ancients the attitudes of all the other organs originate in the energy of the gall bladder. It is different from the other hollow organs in that all the others transport "impure" or foreign matters – food, liquids, and the waste products of these. Only the gall bladder transports "pure" liquids exclusively, in that it stores and concentrates bile.

This meridian is one of the most well-travelled meridians, traversing almost the entire body except the arms. It zigzags throughout the head in a pattern that, in times of stress and tension, becomes like a vice and is, therefore, important in cases of headaches and neck tension.

The *Nei Ching* says that the gall bladder rules decision making, thus anger and rash decisions may be due to an excess of gall bladder ch'i, while indecision may be a sign of gall bladder disharmony and weakness.[11]

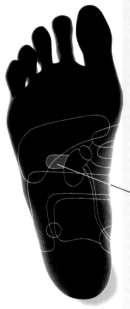

The gall bladder reflex.

Asthma

Shingles

Shoulder pains

Pain in groin region

Arthritic pain in hip

Temple migraines

Skin problems along the meridian (e.g. varicose veins or psoriasis)

Eye weakness, pains lateral to the eye

Ear weakness

Knee complaints (lateral side)

Neck tension

Corns (fourth toe), athlete's foot (fourth toe), hammertoe

THE GALL BLADDER MERIDIAN STARTS AT THE OUTER CORNER OF THE EYE, CROSSES THE TEMPLE AND DESCENDS TO THE SHOULDER. IT CONTINUES LATERALLY DOWN THE BODY AND LEG TO END ON THE BACK OF THE FOURTH TOE TOWARD THE LITTLE TOE.

10 – VEITH P133   11 – TED J. KAPTCHUK, O.M.D. "THE WEB THAT HAS NO WEAVER" PP66–67

LIVER MERIDIAN

The liver rules following and spreading, according to the Chinese classics. The liver or liver ch'i is responsible for the smooth movement of bodily substances and for the regularity of body activities. It moves the ch'i and blood in all directions, sending them to every part of the body. The *Nei Ching* metaphorically calls the liver "the general of an army" because it maintains evenness and harmony of movement throughout the body.[12]

The liver is the primary center of metabolism. Not only does it secrete bile, synthesize proteins, neutralize toxins, and regulate blood sugar levels, it also stores glycogen (starch), changes it back into glucose (sugar), and releases it when needed. Since the brain does not store any glucose, the liver's steady supply is crucial to life, and this is why the Chinese saw the liver as vital to conscious and unconscious thought processes.

The liver meridian helps control the functions of the nervous system and is important for psychological problems such as depression and anger. Motivation – the will to become "that self which one truly is" – is associated with the balance of this meridian along with a sense of well-being and a reasonable temperament.

YIN MERIDIAN

PARTNER MERIDIAN: GALL BLADDER - YANG

ELEMENT: WOOD

ORGAN MAXIMUM ENERGY PERIOD: 1A.M. TO 3A.M.

Liver problems (right side), stomach/spleen problems (left side)

Digestive problems

Eczema, genital problems in males and females, e.g. herpes, low sperm count, impotence, low sexual libido, candida

Eczema or psoriasis along meridian

Thigh pain, varicose veins

Shinbone sores and phlebitis

Problems in big toe, e.g. gout, ingrowing toenail, fungus, corns

Knee pain (medial side)

THE LIVER MERIDIAN STARTS AT THE BACK OF THE BIG TOE AND ASCENDS IMMEDIATELY UP THE LEG TO THE GENITAL REGION AND CONTINUES UPWARD TO JUST BELOW THE NIPPLE ON THE LOWER PART OF THE BREASTBONE.

8. MAPPING THE REFLEXES ON THE FEET

The first and most important step to a full understanding of reflexology techniques is an appreciation of the structure of the feet and how they relate to the body. This is, in fact, simple since the feet are a microcosm or minimap of the whole body, and all the organs and body parts are reflected on the feet as reflex areas in an arrangement similar to their position in the body.

RIGHT
The body is divided into four horizontal zones. These areas are clearly delineated on the soles of the feet.

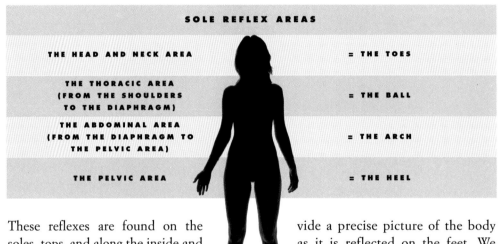

SOLE REFLEX AREAS	
THE HEAD AND NECK AREA	= THE TOES
THE THORACIC AREA (FROM THE SHOULDERS TO THE DIAPHRAGM)	= THE BALL
THE ABDOMINAL AREA (FROM THE DIAPHRAGM TO THE PELVIC AREA)	= THE ARCH
THE PELVIC AREA	= THE HEEL

These reflexes are found on the soles, tops, and along the inside and outside of the feet. Their positions follow a logical anatomical pattern and are clearly related to the meridians we have just looked at.

The body itself is divided horizontally into four parts. These areas can be clearly delineated on the feet, and pro-vide a precise picture of the body as it is reflected on the feet. We will, therefore, examine the situation of body organs in horizontal divisions for ease of study and reference, and to fit in more accurately with the massage technique I teach. This is easiest to understand if studied together with the meridians.

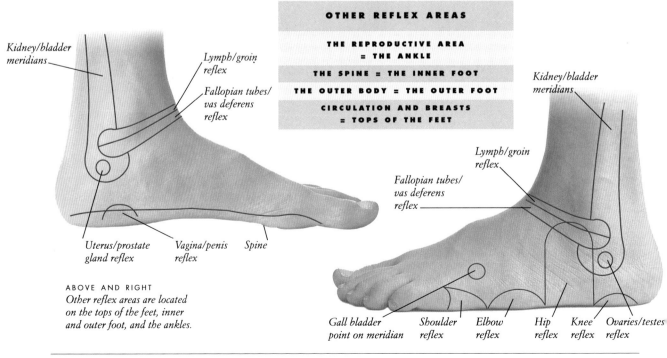

OTHER REFLEX AREAS
THE REPRODUCTIVE AREA = THE ANKLE
THE SPINE = THE INNER FOOT
THE OUTER BODY = THE OUTER FOOT
CIRCULATION AND BREASTS = TOPS OF THE FEET

Kidney/bladder meridians
Lymph/groin reflex
Fallopian tubes/ vas deferens reflex
Uterus/prostate gland reflex
Vagina/penis reflex
Spine

Kidney/bladder meridians
Lymph/groin reflex
Fallopian tubes/ vas deferens reflex
Gall bladder point on meridian
Shoulder reflex
Elbow reflex
Hip reflex
Knee reflex
Ovaries/testes reflex

ABOVE AND RIGHT
Other reflex areas are located on the tops of the feet, inner and outer foot, and the ankles.

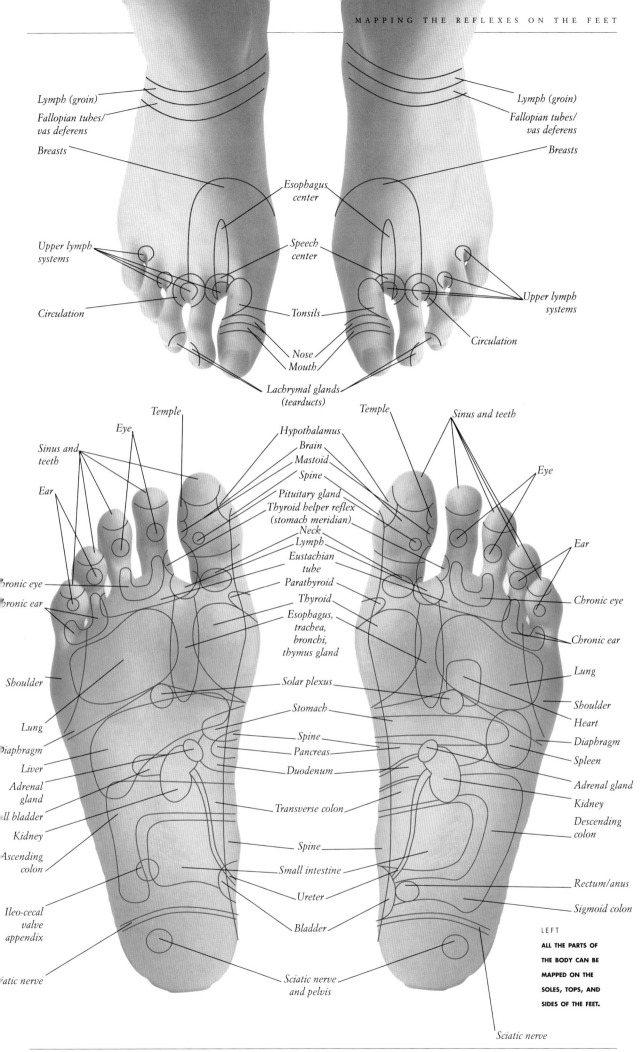

Lymph (groin)
Fallopian tubes/ vas deferens
Breasts
Esophagus center
Speech center
Upper lymph systems
Circulation
Tonsils
Nose
Mouth
Lachrymal glands (tearducts)

Lymph (groin)
Fallopian tubes/ vas deferens
Breasts
Upper lymph systems
Circulation

Temple
Eye
Sinus and teeth
Ear
Chronic eye
Chronic ear
Shoulder
Lung
Diaphragm
Liver
Adrenal gland
Gall bladder
Kidney
Ascending colon
Ileo-cecal valve appendix
Sciatic nerve

Hypothalamus
Brain
Mastoid
Spine
Pituitary gland
Thyroid helper reflex (stomach meridian)
Neck
Lymph
Eustachian tube
Parathyroid
Thyroid
Esophagus, trachea, bronchi, thymus gland
Solar plexus
Stomach
Spine
Pancreas
Duodenum
Transverse colon
Spine
Small intestine
Ureter
Bladder
Sciatic nerve and pelvis

Temple
Sinus and teeth
Eye
Ear
Chronic eye
Chronic ear
Lung
Shoulder
Heart
Diaphragm
Spleen
Adrenal gland
Kidney
Descending colon
Rectum/anus
Sigmoid colon

LEFT
ALL THE PARTS OF
THE BODY CAN BE
MAPPED ON THE
SOLES, TOPS, AND
SIDES OF THE FEET.

Sciatic nerve

The Head and Neck Area – the Toes

BELOW
The toes contain reflexes for all parts of the body above the shoulder li

The toes incorporate reflexes to all parts of the body found above the shoulder girdle. If you imagine the two big toes as two half heads with a common neck, the positions of the reflexes are placed logically. Each big toe contains reflex points for the pituitary gland, pineal gland, hypothalamus, brain, temples, teeth, the seven cervical (neck) vertebrae, sinuses, mastoids, tonsils, nose, mouth, and other face reflexes as well as part of the Eustachian tubes.

The other four toes on each foot contain reflex points for the eyes, ears, teeth, sinuses, lachrymal glands (tearducts), speech center, upper lymph system, collar bone (shoulder girdle), Eustachian tubes, chronic eyes and ears.

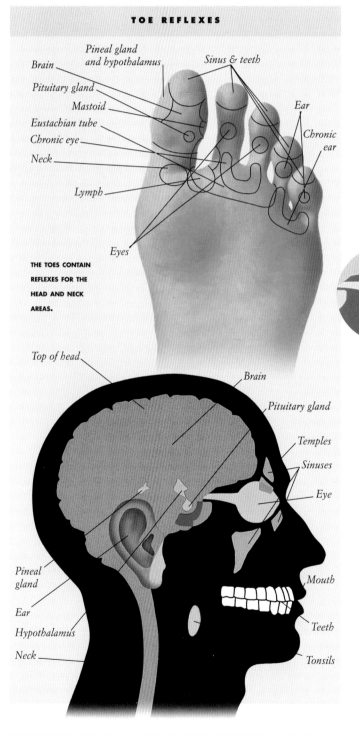

TOE REFLEXES

THE TOES CONTAIN REFLEXES FOR THE HEAD AND NECK AREAS.

THE HEAD AND THE BRAIN

Reflexes of the head and the brain are on the pads of the big toes from the tip behind the nail down over the metatarsal bone; reflexes for the sides of the head and brain are on the sides of the big toes. On the top of the toes are the face reflexes including the mouth, nose, teeth, and tonsils. At the base of each big toe are the neck reflexes.

SINUSES

The sinuses are cavities within the skull bones situated above and to the sides of the nose, in the cheekbones and behind the eyebrows.

THE PITUITARY GLAND

This gland, known also as the "master gland," is considered the most important in the body because it controls the functions of all the endocrine glands. About the size and shape of a cherry, the pituitary gland is attached to the base of the brain. Numerous hormones are produced by the pituitary gland – these influence growth, sexual development, metabolism, pregnancy, mineral and sugar content of the blood, fluid retention, and also influence energy levels.

The reflex point is found on both feet where the whorl of the toe print converges into a central point. It is usually situated on the inner side of the toe.

THE HYPOTHALAMUS

This part of the brain regulates the autonomic nervous system and controls emotional reactions, appetite, body temperature, and also sleep.

The reflex areas are found on both feet on the outer side and top of the big toe.

THE PINEAL GLAND

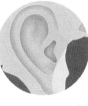

The pineal gland is a small gland situated within the hypothalamus section of the brain. It is known to stimulate the cells in the skin to produce the black pigment melanin. It is thought to play a part in mood and also in circadian rhythms.

The reflexes are on both feet on the outer tip of the big toes – the same as the hypothalamus reflex.

THE TEETH

The reflexes to the teeth are exactly distributed over the ten toes: incisors on the big toe; incisors and canine teeth on the second toe; premolars on the third toe; molars on the fourth toe; wisdom teeth on the fifth toe. These reflexes are in the same position as the sinus reflexes.

THE EYES

The eyes are important sensory organs – the organs of sight. These reflexes are on both feet on the cushions of the second and third toes and may extend slightly down on the toes. Reflexes for chronic eye conditions are on the "shelf" at the base of these two toes.

THE EARS

The ear is the organ of hearing. It also plays an important part in maintaining the body's balance.

The reflexes are situated on both feet on the cushions of the fourth and fifth toes and may extend slightly down the toes. The reflexes for the Eustachian tubes extend from the inner side of the big toe along the base of the second and third toes to the fourth toe. Reflexes for chronic ear conditions are found on the "shelf" at the base of these two toes – the same section as the Eustachian tubes. The mastoid – the part of the skull behind the ear containing the air spaces that communicate with the ear – is also treated on these reflexes.

THE TONSILS

These are paired organs that defend the throat area. The reflexes are found on both feet – on the top of the foot at the base of the big toe near the web between the big and second toes.

THE LYMPHATIC SYSTEM

The lymphatic system is a network of lymphatic vessels situated at various sites throughout the body. Lymph nodes filter the lymph to prevent infection from passing into the bloodstream and add lymphocytes, which are important in the body's immune system for the formation of antibodies and immunological reactions. The main sites of the lymph nodes are in the neck, armpits, breasts, abdomen, groin, pelvis, and behind the knees.

On the front of the foot, in the webs between the toes are the reflexes for lymph drainage in the neck and chest region of the body. Lymph reflexes for the groin area are linked to the reproductive system and run across the top of the foot from the inner ankle bone to the outer ankle bone. These lymph reflexes also incorporate the six main meridians.

The Thoracic Area – the Ball of the Foot

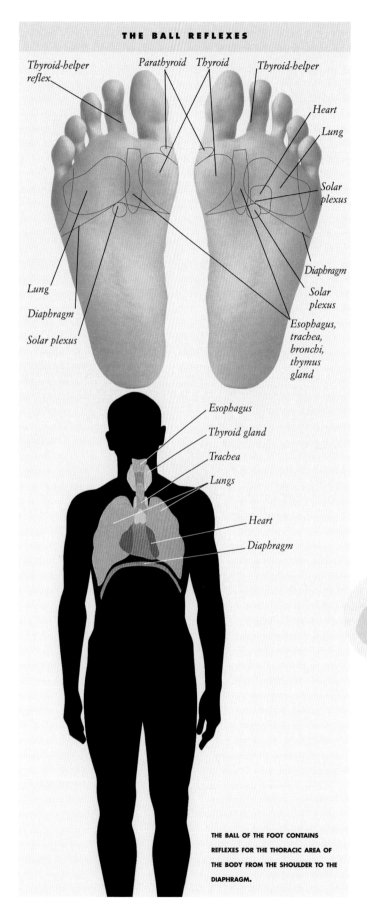

THE BALL REFLEXES

Thyroid-helper reflex

Parathyroid

Thyroid

Thyroid-helper

Heart

Lung

Solar plexus

Lung

Diaphragm

Solar plexus

Diaphragm

Solar plexus

Esophagus, trachea, bronchi, thymus gland

Esophagus

Thyroid gland

Trachea

Lungs

Heart

Diaphragm

THE BALL OF THE FOOT CONTAINS REFLEXES FOR THE THORACIC AREA OF THE BODY FROM THE SHOULDER TO THE DIAPHRAGM.

This section of the foot corresponds with the thoracic area in the body from the shoulder girdle to the diaphragm. Several vital reflexes are situated here: the heart, lungs, esophagus, trachea, bronchi, thyroid and thymus glands, diaphragm, and solar plexus.

THE LUNGS

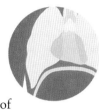

The lungs are cone-shaped, spongy organs that lie in the thorax on either side of the heart. It is here that the process of respiration takes place – the exchange of oxygen for carbon dioxide. The air passages of the respiratory system found in the thorax are the trachea (windpipe), which divides into the bronchi to enter the left and right lungs.

The lung reflexes are found on the soles of both feet from the second toe (stomach meridian) to just past the fourth toe (gall bladder meridian). Reflexes for the trachea and bronchi are found below the big toe and second toe (stomach and liver meridians) connected to the lung reflex. These same reflexes are also found in similar positions on the tops of the feet.

THE HEART

The heart is a hollow, cone-shaped, muscular organ that lies in the chest on the left side of the body inside the rib cage in a space between the lungs. It acts as a pump circulating blood throughout the body. Efficient functioning of the heart is essential to allow good blood circulation, which is necessary for efficient transportation of gases, foods, and waste products. The chest area also contains other major vessels leading to and from the heart – the arteries, veins, venae cavae, and aorta.

The reflex to the heart is situated on the sole of the left foot only – on the kidney meridian above the diaphragm level in the center of the ball area.

THE THYMUS GLAND, ESOPHAGUS, TRACHEA, AND BRONCHI

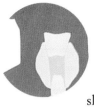

The thymus gland is situated in the thoracic cavity. It is quite large in childhood, reaches maximum size at 10 to 12, then slowly regresses and almost disappears in adult life. It is involved in the immune system, but its only known function is the formation of lymphocytes – white cells in the blood.

The esophagus is the gullet – a muscular tube passing from the pharynx down through the chest and joining the stomach below the diaphragm. Food and fluid are propelled through it by peristalsis, the wavelike contractions occurring in the intestinal walls.

The trachea is the windpipe. It passes down from the larynx into the chest where it divides into two bronchi, the main diversions of the trachea that enter the lungs.

All these reflexes are found on both feet in the same area – on the soles of the feet in a vertical band between the first and second toes.

THE THYROID GLAND

The thyroid gland is located in the neck. It secretes thyroxin, a hormone that influences all the major systems of the body. The thyroid gland controls the rate of metabolism and maintains the correct amount of calcium circulating in the blood.

This reflex is situated on both feet on the lower crease at the base of the big toe, down around the ball and into the groove below the bone. Half is found on each foot on the inner edge. The most important part is the section situated along the bone itself.

There is also a "helper" reflex on the second toe – the stomach meridian.

THE PARATHYROID GLANDS

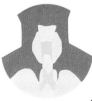

These are four small glands situated around the thyroid gland. Their main function is to maintain the correct amount of the minerals, calcium, and phosphorus in the blood and bones.

The parathyroid gland reflex is situated on both feet at the base of the big toe on the inner edge of the foot.

THE DIAPHRAGM

The diaphragm, one of the muscles of respiration, is a large, dome-shaped wall that separates the thorax from the abdomen. It is the most important muscle required for breathing.

This reflex is situated on the soles of both feet, extends across all six meridians at the base of the ball of the foot separating the ball from the arch.

THE SOLAR PLEXUS

The solar plexus is a network of sympathetic nerve ganglia in the abdomen and is the nerve supply to the abdominal organs below the diaphragm. Sometimes called the "abdominal brain" or the "nerve switchboard," it is situated behind the stomach and in front of the diaphragm.

The reflex is immediately below the ball of the foot at the same level as the reflex to the diaphragm, located at a specific point in the center of the diaphragm reflex. This point is visible on the foot as the apex of the arch that runs across the base of the ball of the foot. Massage on this reflex can relieve stress and nervousness, aid deep regular breathing, and restore calm. Particularly beneficial to those with nervous disorders, allergies, asthma, or skin irritations, massage of this reflex has even been shown to help young children to sleep!

The Abdominal Area – the Arch of the Foot

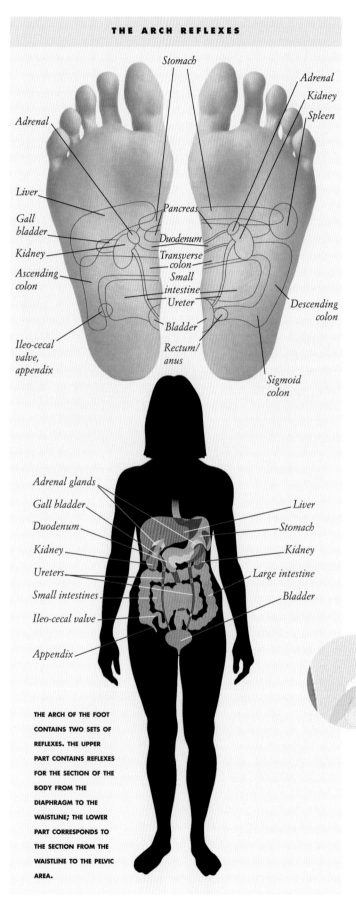

THE ARCH REFLEXES

Stomach

Adrenal
Kidney
Spleen

Adrenal

Liver

Gall bladder

Kidney

Ascending colon

Ileo-cecal valve, appendix

Pancreas

Duodenum

Transverse colon

Small intestine

Ureter

Bladder

Rectum/anus

Descending colon

Sigmoid colon

Adrenal glands

Gall bladder

Duodenum

Kidney

Ureters

Small intestines

Ileo-cecal valve

Appendix

Liver

Stomach

Kidney

Large intestine

Bladder

THE ARCH OF THE FOOT CONTAINS TWO SETS OF REFLEXES. THE UPPER PART CONTAINS REFLEXES FOR THE SECTION OF THE BODY FROM THE DIAPHRAGM TO THE WAISTLINE; THE LOWER PART CORRESPONDS TO THE SECTION FROM THE WAISTLINE TO THE PELVIC AREA.

The arch of the foot is clearly visible on the sole – the raised area that extends from the base of the ball to the beginning of the heel. It is divided into two parts: the upper part corresponds to the section of the body from the diaphragm to the waistline; the lower part corresponds to the section of the body from the waistline to the pelvic area.

Reflexes above the waistline are the: liver, gall bladder, stomach, pancreas, duodenum, spleen, adrenals, and kidneys.

THE LIVER

The liver is the largest and most complex organ/gland in the body. It controls many of the body's chemical processes and has many functions. These include: processing nutrients from the blood; storing fats and proteins until the body needs them; detoxifying the blood and manufacturing bile for fat digestion; storing glucose sugars in the form of glycogen to be used when the body needs to draw on an increased supply of energy.

The liver reflex is found on the sole of the right foot only, below the diaphragm level, extending from the spleen/pancreas meridian on the inside of the foot to below the little toe. The reflex ends just above the waistline area on the foot.

THE GALL BLADDER

This is a small, muscular, pear-shaped sac attached to the undersurface of the liver. Its function is to excrete bile for the digestion of food.

The gall bladder reflex is on the sole of the right foot only, embedded within the liver reflex, beneath and between the third and fourth toes.

THE STOMACH

The stomach is a large, muscular sac that lies

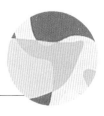

below the diaphragm mainly to the left side of the body.

The reflexes are found on the soles of both feet – extending from the big toe to the outer edge of the fourth toe on the left foot. Horizontally, they are situated just below the diaphragm level.

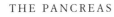

THE PANCREAS

The pancreas is a large glandular structure in the abdomen. It is probably best known for the production of the hormones insulin and glucagon.

The reflexes are situated on the soles of both feet – more on the left foot than the right foot – below the stomach and above the waistline. On the right foot it extends to just below the big toe, and on the left foot as far as the fourth toe.

THE DUODENUM

This is the first, C-shaped part of the small intestine, that is about 8 to 10 in. long. Pancreatic and common bile ducts open into it, releasing secretions that are responsible for the breakdown of food.

The reflexes are on the soles of both feet immediately below the pancreas, touching the waistline and extending inward to the second toe.

THE SPLEEN

The spleen is a large, vascular, gland-like but ductless organ found on the left side of the body behind the stomach. It contains lymphatic tissue that manufactures the white blood cells, breaks down old red blood corpuscles and filters toxins from the lymph.

The spleen reflex is found on the outer side of the left foot (opposite the liver reflex on the right foot), beneath the

fourth toe (gall bladder meridian) and just below the diaphragm, in a direct line with the stomach reflex.

THE KIDNEYS

The kidneys are part of the main excretory system of the body – the urinary system – which collectively refers to the kidneys, ureter tubes, urethra, and bladder. They are two bean-shaped organs that filter toxins from the blood, produce urine, and regulate the retention of important minerals and water.

The reflexes are found on the soles of both feet, positioned just above the waistline on the kidney and stomach meridians, just below the stomach reflex. The right kidney is positioned slightly lower than the left kidney.

THE ADRENAL GLANDS

These are two triangular endocrine glands situated on the upper tip of each kidney. The adrenal glands are divided into two distinct regions, the cortex and medulla. The adrenal cortex produces steroid hormones that regulate carbohydrate metabolism and have antiallergic and antiinflammatory properties. The cortex also produces hormones that control the reabsorption of sodium and water in the kidneys, as well as the secretion of potassium and the sex hormones testosterone, estrogen, and progesterone. The adrenal medulla produce adrenalin and noradrenalin, which work in conjunction with the sympathetic nervous system. The output of adrenalin is increased at times of anxiety and stress when the body needs to prepare for "fight-or-flight" *(see pages 22–23).*

The reflexes for the adrenal glands are situated on the soles of both feet immediately above the area of the kidney reflexes. They occupy the area toward the center of the arch of the foot.

THE SMALL INTESTINE

This is a muscular tube about 20 to 23ft. in length and is the main area of the digestive tract where absorption takes place. It lies in a coiled position in the abdominal cavity surrounded by the large intestine. The small intestine is divided into three sections – these are the duodenum, jejunum, and the ileum.

The reflex is situated on the soles of both feet, under the large intestine reflex, extending horizontally across the arch to below the fourth toe.

THE ILEO-CECAL VALVE

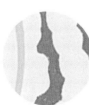

The ileo-cecal valve is situated at the point where the small intestine and large intestine join, and therefore controls the passage of contents of the small intestine through to the large intestine. It prevents back-flow of fecal matter from the large intestine and controls mucous secretions.

The reflex for the ileo-cecal valve is found on the sole of the right foot below and between the third and fourth toes, just above the level of the pelvic floor.

THE APPENDIX

The appendix is a worm-like tube about 3 to 4 in. in length, with a blind end projecting. Located directly below the ileo-cecal valve, it helps to lubricate the large intestine, is rich in lymphoid tissue, and secretes antibodies into the bloodstream.

The appendix reflex is situated on the sole of the right foot only, in the same area as the ileo-cecal valve.

THE LARGE INTESTINE

The large intestine is a tube about 5ft. in length that surrounds the small intestine. The tube starts on the right side of the body, goes up the right side to below the liver where it bends to the left (hepatic flexure) and passes across the abdomen as the transverse colon. At the left side of the abdomen, it bends down below the spleen (splenic flexure) to become the descending colon, which passes down the left side of the abdomen. The tube then turns toward the midline and takes the shape of a double S-shaped bend known as the sigmoid flexure. This leads into the rectum and then, the anus.

The reflexes for the large intestine are found on the soles of both feet. On the right foot this begins just below the reflex for the ileo-cecal valve and extends upward (ascending colon), turns just below the liver reflex to become the transverse colon, which extends across the entire foot. It continues across to the left foot and turns just below the spleen reflex to become the descending colon. Just above the pelvic floor it turns again into the sigmoid colon, which ends at the reflex of the rectum/anus.

THE URETERS

The ureters are muscular tubes about 12 in. in length, which connect the kidneys and bladder. The ureters function as a passageway for urine. There are two tubes, one from each kidney, which pass downward through the abdomen into the pelvis where they enter the bladder.

The reflexes for the ureters are narrow strips situated on the soles of both feet. They link the kidney reflexes to the bladder reflexes.

THE BLADDER

The bladder is an elastic muscular sac situated in the center of the pelvis. Urine for excretion passes from the kidneys down the ureters and is stored in the bladder until it is eliminated via the urethra. The reflexes are found on both feet, on the side of the foot below the inner ankle bone on the heel line.

The Pelvic Area – the Heel of the Foot

Few organs are represented here, but this area is of vital importance since all six main meridians traverse the pelvic section of the heel. As a result, many congestions here can be traced to meridians and their corresponding organs.

THE SCIATIC NERVES

The sciatic nerves are the largest nerves in the body measuring 0.8 in. across at the start. They arise from the sacral plexus of nerves formed by the lower lumbar and upper sacral spinal nerves. They run from the buttocks in a broad band down the backs of the thighs to divide just above the knees into two main branches called the tibial and common peroneal nerves, which supply the lower legs. These are actual nerves in the feet and are also reflex areas.

Sciatica is a common ailment affecting the sciatic nerves. It is characterized by a sharp, stabbing pain down the back of the leg, along the sciatic nerve from the buttocks to the ankle. Sciatica is often caused by vertebrae pressing on the nerve.

The sciatic nerves and reflexes are found on the soles of both feet, in a band about a third of the way down the pad of the heel extending across the floor.

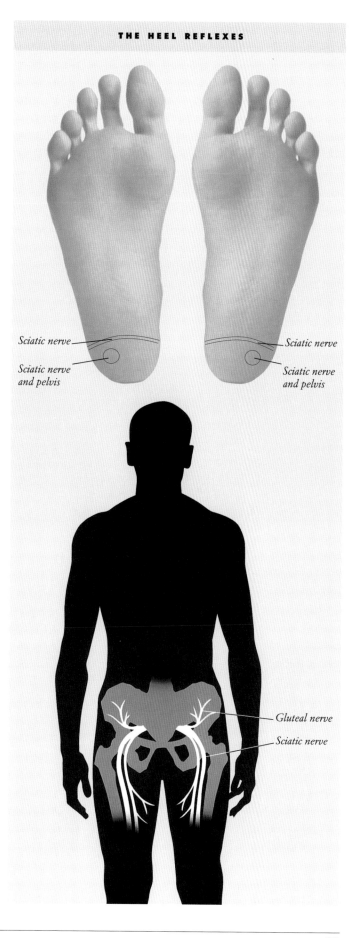

THE HEEL REFLEXES

Sciatic nerve
Sciatic nerve and pelvis
Sciatic nerve
Sciatic nerve and pelvis

Gluteal nerve
Sciatic nerve

RIGHT
THE HEEL OF THE FOOT
CONTAINS THE REFLEXES
FOR THE SCIATIC NERVES,
THE LARGEST NERVES IN
THE BODY.

The Reproductive Area – the Ankle

BELOW

THE ANKLE AREA
CONTAINS THE
REPRODUCTIVE ORGAN
REFLEXES FOR BOTH
MALES AND FEMALES.
THE UTERUS/ PROSTATE
GLAND AND VAGINA/
PENIS REFLEXES ARE
FOUND ONLY ON THE
INNER ANKLE. THE
OVARIES/TESTES REFLEX
IS FOUND ONLY ON THE
OUTER ANKLE.

The outer ankle contains the ovaries/testes reflexes, and the inner ankle contains reflexes of the uterus, prostate, vagina, and penis. The reflex points for the Fallopian tubes, lymph drainage area in the groin, vas deferens, and seminal vesicles are found in a narrow band running below the outer ankle bone across the top of the foot to the inner ankle bone. The kidney/bladder meridian is situated on both sides of the back of the Achilles tendon.

The ovaries are the female gonads or sex glands. The reflexes are found on both feet on the outer side, midway between the ankle bone and the back of the heel – the right ovary on the right foot, the left ovary on the left foot. The "helper" area is the heel due to the presence of the meridians.

The testes are the male reproductive glands. The reflexes are found on males in the same area as the ovaries in females – midway between the outer ankle bone and the heel. The "helper" area is the heel.

The uterus is a hollow pear-shaped organ about 4 in. long, situated in the center of the pelvic cavity in females. The reflex points are located on both feet on the inside of the ankles, midway on a diagonal line between the ankle bone and the back of the heel. As with the ovaries and testes, the "helper" area is the heel.

The prostate gland lies at the base of the bladder in males and surrounds the urethra. Reflexes are found on both feet in the same place as the uterus reflex on females – midway in a diagonal line between the inner ankle bone and the heel. Again, the heel is the "helper" area.

In females the Fallopian tubes, two tubes about 4 to 5 in. in length, connect the ovaries with the cavity of the uterus. Their function is to conduct the ova expelled from the ovaries during ovulation down to the uterus.

The Fallopian tube reflexes are found on both feet. They run across the top of the foot linking the reflex of the uterus to the reflex of the ovaries. This area is usually massaged in conjunction with the reflexes of the ovaries and uterus.

In males the seminal vesicles lie next to the prostate and store semen. The vas deferens are a pair of excretory ducts that are designed to convey semen from the testes to the urethra.

The reflexes for the seminal vesicles and vas deferens are located in the same area as the Fallopian tubes in females – across the top of the foot from one ankle bone to the other, linking the prostate and testes reflexes.

THE ANKLE REFLEXES

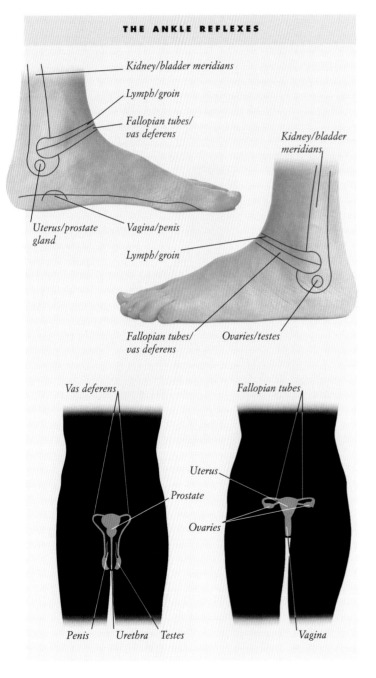

Kidney/bladder meridians

Lymph/groin

Fallopian tubes/ vas deferens

Kidney/bladder meridians

Uterus/prostate gland

Vagina/penis

Lymph/groin

Fallopian tubes/ vas deferens

Ovaries/testes

Vas deferens

Fallopian tubes

Uterus

Prostate

Ovaries

Penis   Urethra   Testes

Vagina

The Spine – the Inner Foot

The inside of each foot is naturally curved to correspond to the spine.

The spine (backbone or vertebral column) is the central support of the body. It carries the weight of the body and is an important axis of movement. It is made up of 33 vertebrae. The structure of the bones is arranged in such a way as to give the spine four curves. The spine is divided into five sections from top to bottom:

* **7 CERVICAL VERTEBRAE (INCLUDING THE AXIS AND ATLAS) = THE NECK**

* **12 THORACIC VERTEBRAE = THE BACK**

* **5 LUMBAR VERTEBRAE = THE LOIN**

* **5 SACRAL VERTEBRAE = THE PELVIS**

* **4 COCCYGEAL VERTEBRAE = THE TAIL**

At the base of the spine the vertebrae of the sacrum and coccyx are fused to form two immobile bones. Vertebrae are joined together by disks of cartilage and are held in place by ligaments.

The spinal column encloses the spinal cord, the central channel of the nervous system, which is a continuation of the brain stem. It carries the nerves from the brain to all parts of the body. Associated with each vertebra is a pair of spinal nerves. These nerves arise from the spinal cord and affect the level of the body at which they arise – thoracic nerves affect the thorax, lumbar nerves the lower abdomen and legs. These nerves supply specific organs so any constriction or damage to them will directly affect the connected body parts. The nerve connections of these vertebrae to the tissue, glands and organs are illustrated above.

The spine reflex runs along the inner side of both feet – half the spine being represented on each foot. The cervical vertebrae reflex runs from the base of the big toenail to the base of the toe (between the first and second joints of the big toe). The thoracic reflex runs along the ball of the foot below the big toe (shoulder to waistline), the arch from the waistline to pelvic line corresponds to the lumbar region, and the heel line to the base of the heel to the sacrum/coccyx.

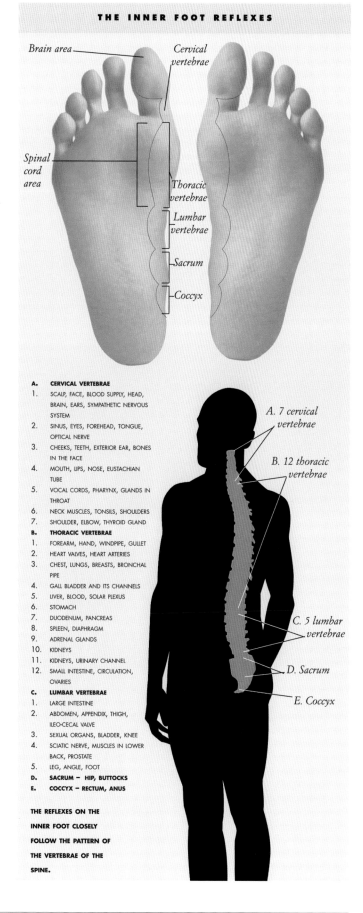

THE INNER FOOT REFLEXES

Brain area

Cervical vertebrae

Spinal cord area

Thoracic vertebrae

Lumbar vertebrae

Sacrum

Coccyx

A. CERVICAL VERTEBRAE
1. SCALP, FACE, BLOOD SUPPLY, HEAD, BRAIN, EARS, SYMPATHETIC NERVOUS SYSTEM
2. SINUS, EYES, FOREHEAD, TONGUE, OPTICAL NERVE
3. CHEEKS, TEETH, EXTERIOR EAR, BONES IN THE FACE
4. MOUTH, LIPS, NOSE, EUSTACHIAN TUBE
5. VOCAL CORDS, PHARYNX, GLANDS IN THROAT
6. NECK MUSCLES, TONSILS, SHOULDERS
7. SHOULDER, ELBOW, THYROID GLAND

B. THORACIC VERTEBRAE
1. FOREARM, HAND, WINDPIPE, GULLET
2. HEART VALVES, HEART ARTERIES
3. CHEST, LUNGS, BREASTS, BRONCHAL PIPE
4. GALL BLADDER AND ITS CHANNELS
5. LIVER, BLOOD, SOLAR PLEXUS
6. STOMACH
7. DUODENUM, PANCREAS
8. SPLEEN, DIAPHRAGM
9. ADRENAL GLANDS
10. KIDNEYS
11. KIDNEYS, URINARY CHANNEL
12. SMALL INTESTINE, CIRCULATION, OVARIES

C. LUMBAR VERTEBRAE
1. LARGE INTESTINE
2. ABDOMEN, APPENDIX, THIGH, ILEO-CECAL VALVE
3. SEXUAL ORGANS, BLADDER, KNEE
4. SCIATIC NERVE, MUSCLES IN LOWER BACK, PROSTATE
5. LEG, ANGLE, FOOT

D. SACRUM – HIP, BUTTOCKS

E. COCCYX – RECTUM, ANUS

THE REFLEXES ON THE INNER FOOT CLOSELY FOLLOW THE PATTERN OF THE VERTEBRAE OF THE SPINE.

A. 7 cervical vertebrae

B. 12 thoracic vertebrae

C. 5 lumbar vertebrae

D. Sacrum

E. Coccyx

The Outer Body – the Outer Foot

The outer edge of the foot corresponds to the outer part of the body – the joints, ligaments, and surrounding muscles:

* FROM THE BASE OF THE TOE TO THE DIAPHRAGM LINE = SHOULDER AND UPPER ARM

* DIAPHRAGM LINE TO WAISTLINE = ELBOW, FOREARM, WRIST, AND HAND

* WAISTLINE TO END OF HEEL = LEG, KNEE, AND HIP

THE OUTER FOOT REFLEXES

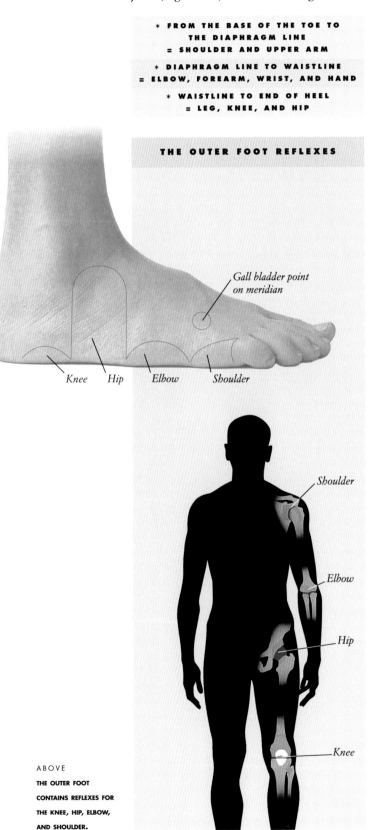

Gall bladder point on meridian

Knee   *Hip*   *Elbow*   *Shoulder*

Shoulder

Elbow

Hip

Knee

ABOVE
THE OUTER FOOT CONTAINS REFLEXES FOR THE KNEE, HIP, ELBOW, AND SHOULDER.

THE KNEE

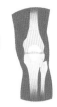

The knee joint joins the upper and lower leg and facilitates movement of the lower part of limb.

Reflexes are found on both feet on the outer side, just below the bony projection of the ankle bone, which is usually quite prominent on the side of the foot.

Again, remember the six meridians run through the knee, so by pinpointing the exact location of the knee pain, one can relate it to a specific meridian and locate the problematic organ.

THE HIP

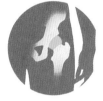

The hip joint is a ball and socket joint where the thigh bone (femur) meets the pelvis.

The reflex is found on both feet extending toward the toe in front of the knee reflex. It covers an oblong shape, moving out from the line up the side of the foot, in line with the fourth toe. A number of hip problems may be gall bladder related, because the gall bladder meridian passes directly through the hip.

THE ELBOW AND SHOULDER

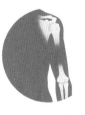

The elbow is the joint between the upper arm and the forearm. It is formed by the humerus above and the radius and ulna below. The shoulder joint is where the bone of the upper arm (humerus) meets the shoulder blade (scapula).

The reflexes to the elbow are situated on both feet on the outer side, along the arch and the ball. Those to the shoulder and the surrounding muscles are found on both feet at the base of the fifth toe covering the sole, outer side, and top of the foot.

The Top of the Foot

Reflexes found on the top of the foot include the circulation and breasts. Most of the reflexes represented on the soles are also found on the top of the feet in the meridians.

BREASTS

If there are breast problems, note exactly where these are so as to identify the meridian that runs through the affected section of the breast and thereby the problem organ.

SPECIAL CIRCULATION POINTS

These special points are to stimulate the heart, circulation, and body temperature. They are situated on the top and soles of both feet at the web between the second and third toes.

Since these are points on the stomach meridian, they have an effect on the thyroid, which in turn controls differences in the level of body temperature, the functioning and speed of the heart, and the body's circulatory system.

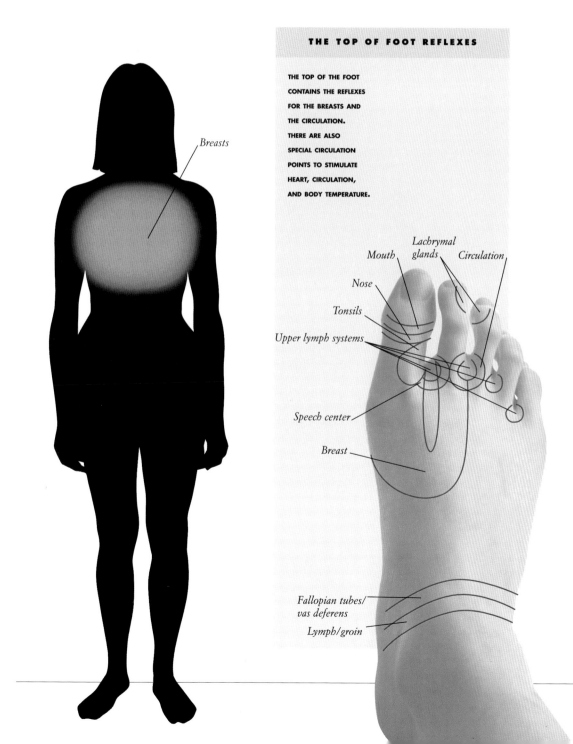

Breasts

THE TOP OF FOOT REFLEXES

THE TOP OF THE FOOT
CONTAINS THE REFLEXES
FOR THE BREASTS AND
THE CIRCULATION.
THERE ARE ALSO
SPECIAL CIRCULATION
POINTS TO STIMULATE
HEART, CIRCULATION,
AND BODY TEMPERATURE.

Mouth

Lachrymal glands

Circulation

Nose

Tonsils

Upper lymph systems

Speech center

Breast

Fallopian tubes/ vas deferens

Lymph/groin

9. INTERPRETING THE FEET

*I*t is estimated that approximately 80 percent of adults will develop foot disorders, even though most people are born with healthy feet. There is a tendency to blame foot problems and deformities – corns, calluses, bunions, and the like – on ill-fitting shoes. This is part of the problem – but only part.

Problem areas on the feet relate to problem areas in the body. Which is the cause and which the effect is questionable; it is a "chicken or egg" situation. Congestions along a meridian or on a reflex – caused by either internal or external factors – will disrupt the body's equilibrium. If the problem is internal, the reflex area and

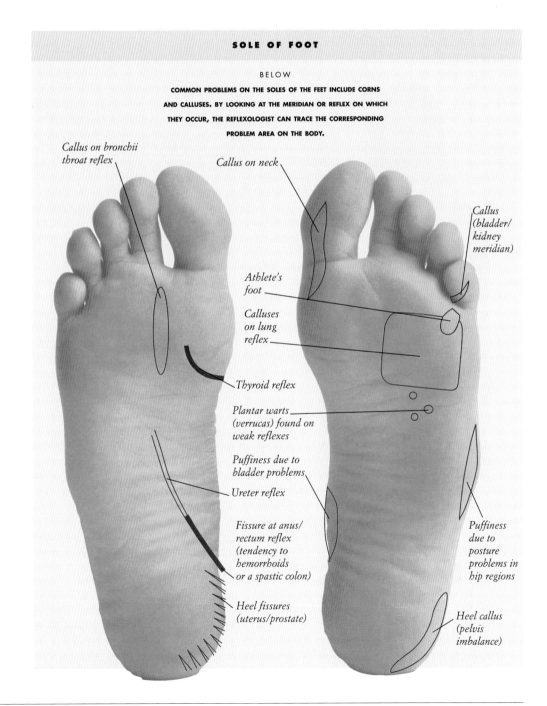

SOLE OF FOOT

BELOW

COMMON PROBLEMS ON THE SOLES OF THE FEET INCLUDE CORNS
AND CALLUSES. BY LOOKING AT THE MERIDIAN OR REFLEX ON WHICH
THEY OCCUR, THE REFLEXOLOGIST CAN TRACE THE CORRESPONDING
PROBLEM AREA ON THE BODY.

Callus on bronchii throat reflex

Callus on neck

Callus (bladder/ kidney meridian)

Athlete's foot

Calluses on lung reflex

Thyroid reflex

Plantar warts (verrucas) found on weak reflexes

Puffiness due to bladder problems

Ureter reflex

Fissure at anus/ rectum reflex (tendency to hemorrhoids or a spastic colon)

Puffiness due to posture problems in hip regions

Heel fissures (uterus/prostate)

Heel callus (pelvis imbalance)

the relevant meridian will be particularly sensitive to excess pressure and friction and more susceptible to the formation of corns, calluses, and other problems.

However, these external problems cause congestions along the meridians in the same way as internal problems. If these meridian congestions are not dealt with they can have an adverse effect on body parts along the entire meridian. This goes on to create imbalance throughout the body. With the combination of reflexes and meridians, we can look at these problems in a different light and unravel the tales they have to tell about the state of the body as a whole. The areas where problems manifest are particularly significant when also taking the meridians into consideration.

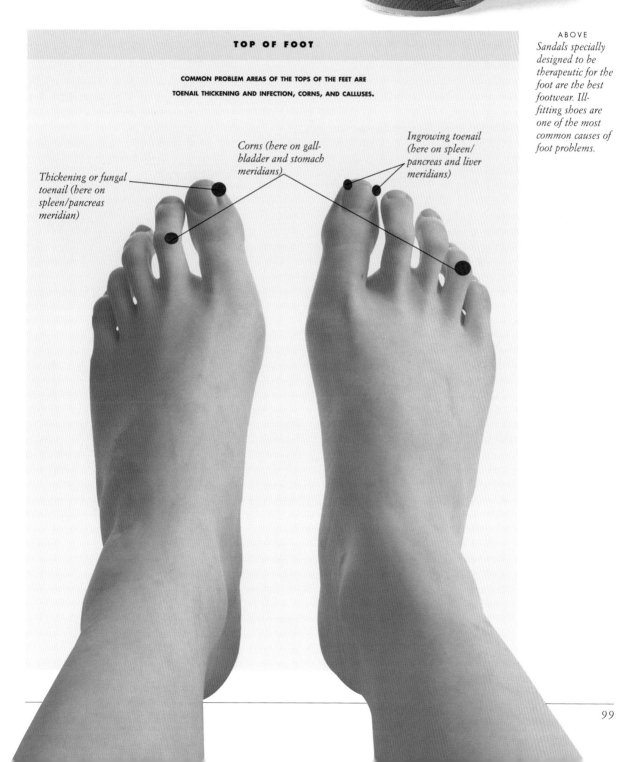

ABOVE
Sandals specially designed to be therapeutic for the foot are the best footwear. Ill-fitting shoes are one of the most common causes of foot problems.

TOP OF FOOT

COMMON PROBLEM AREAS OF THE TOPS OF THE FEET ARE
TOENAIL THICKENING AND INFECTION, CORNS, AND CALLUSES.

Corns (here on gall-bladder and stomach meridians)

Ingrowing toenail (here on spleen/pancreas and liver meridians)

Thickening or fungal toenail (here on spleen/pancreas meridian)

BELOW
This bunion shows how the swelling pushes the big toe out of alignment.

Bone and Joint Problems

BUNIONS (HALLUX VALGUS)

A bunion is a prominence on the head of the metatarsal bone at its junction with the big toe. It is caused by inflammation and swelling of the bursa (bursitis) at that joint. The bursa is a pocket of fluid enclosed in fibrous tissue that surrounds the joints and serves to protect them from friction. In this condition the metatarsal joint becomes enlarged and is therefore subject to pressure and friction from shoes, which further aggravates the problem and damages the skin. Shoes are a major problem in this condition, especially pointed, high-heeled shoes, which thrust the foot forward and exert an enormous amount of pressure on the big toe.

The constriction of the toes can also affect the little toe, forcing it toward the middle of the foot and causing a "bunionette" on the outer side at the base of the little toe. Bunions look and feel unnatural and usually require surgical removal. Barefooted people are less apt to develop bunions.

RIGHT
A red, swollen bunion on this woman's right foot has forced the big toe to overlap the second toe.

ABOVE
A bunion on a woman's right foot, caused by wearing ill-fitting shoes or an imbalance on the spleen/pancreas meridian.

BUNIONS AND HAMMERTOES ARE COMMONLY CAUSED BY ILL-FITTING SHOES, BUT RIGID TOE IS USUALLY THE RESULT OF INJURY OR ARTHRITIS.

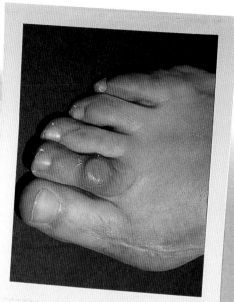

ABOVE
This adult's second toe displays the classic features of hammertoe. The patient has a corn on the hammertoe where it rubs against shoes.

HAMMERTOE

This condition often accompanies bunions. It occurs when the medial joints bend so that the toe rises above the other toes and the top joint is almost curled under. Tendons and ligaments contract to such an extent that they pull the front of the toe backward. This affliction is most common on the second toe.

High-arched feet are more inclined to develop hammertoes because of the positioning of the ligaments. Shoes aggravate this condition. With age, hammertoes may become more rigid and require surgery to correct.

RIGID TOE (HALLUX RIGIDUS)

A rigid toe can be the result of osteoarthritis, injury, obesity, or flat feet. The big toe fuses with the metatarsal bone and creates unnatural stiffness. Walking becomes a problem because the big toe has lost its flexibility. As the range of motion decreases, damage mounts. Joint replacement may be the only answer.

BELOW
Arthritis in the joints of the big toe has caused this hallux rigidus.

ABOVE
Rigid toe is often the result of flat feet – the big toe is unnaturally stiff.

101

RIGHT
*This ankle deformed by
rheumatoid arthritis is also
affected by cellulitis, a
bacterial infection of the
skin and underlying tissue.*

ARTHRITIS

There are many types of
arthritis – some due to
infection, others due to
trauma. Arthritis causes
cartilage to degenerate and
the bones to become over-
grown or waste away. In most
cases it attacks the linings of
joints, which then become stiff,
swollen, and painful. Muscles that
move joints are unable to work correctly, so waste away. Tissues around
the joints become inflamed, filled with
fluid, and painful.

RIGHT
*Rheumatoid
arthritis has
caused this foot
deformity,
damaging the toe
joints and
surrounding
tissues.*

The two common strains of arthritis
are osteoarthritis and rheumatoid arthritis. Osteoarthritis is a degenerative condition attacking the protective cartilage
around the bone ends and is aggravated
by an impaired blood supply, previous
injury, or being overweight. It mainly
affects the weight-bearing joints.

Rheumatoid arthritis is a chronic
inflammation, usually of unknown origin.
The disease is progressive and incapaci-
tating. This condition usually affects the
elderly and is more common among
women than men. It could be a virus
infection and is often triggered by emotional stress. Patients suffering from
rheumatoid arthritis are more susceptible
to infection because arthritis is an auto-
immune disorder.

GOUT

Gout is a metabolic disease associated with an excess of uric acid
in the blood. It is characterized
by painful inflammation and swelling of
the smaller joints, and generally favors
the big toe. Inflammation is accompanied
by the deposit of urates around the joints.
This condition mostly affects males, and
there is a possibility that it is triggered by
emotional stress.

RIGHT
*The joints of these
toes are swollen and
inflamed because of
gout, an
accumulation of uric
acid salts in the
blood circulation
and joints.*

**ARTHRITIS AND GOUT
CAN CAUSE SEVERE
BONE AND JOINT
DISORDERS IN THE FEET.**

MERIDIANS AND
BONE/JOINT PROBLEMS

Two important meridians are found on the big toe – the spleen/pancreas meridian on the outer side, and the liver meridian on the inner side toward the second toe. Bunions are situated on the pancreas meridian and the thyroid reflex. The internal branch of the spleen/pancreas meridian runs through the thyroid, further indicating their close relationship. Most people with bunions also have problems along the spleen/pancreas meridian or pancreatic disorders, such as problems related to sugar metabolism such as a sweet tooth; cravings for stimulants such as tea, coffee, cigarettes, and alcohol; and constant hunger. They may suffer from depression due to the fact that the thyroid is affected. Many people who have had bunions removed or repaired at an early age often develop thyroid problems in later life. Or vice versa – people with thyroid problems often develop bunions. This is because the underlying causes of the symptom – pancreas and thyroid imbalance – have not been corrected.

Once a bunion has developed in an adult foot it cannot be realigned or straightened without surgery. No exercise or manipulation will push it back. By understanding the connection with the meridians, we can understand the cause of the problem – a pancreas imbalance – and set about rectifying that. This problem is most effectively rectified by a change of diet. Pain caused by bunions can be significantly alleviated with reflexology treatments and a change of diet.

In the condition of a hammertoe, relate where it appears to a meridian. It often occurs on the second toe (stomach meridian) or the fourth toe (gall bladder meridian), and other symptoms may be related to imbalance along these meridians. The rigid toe manifests on the big toe and therefore relates to the spleen/pancreas and liver meridians.

MERIDIANS, REFLEXES,
ARTHRITIS, AND GOUT

Since gout favors the big toe, this can be related to the spleen/pancreas and liver meridians, indicating problems with overacid diet. The other forms of arthritis may manifest anywhere in the foot joints; relate this to refle-xes and meridians for further insight into the problem organ. By increasing blood flow to the feet, reflexology can help alleviate the pain and encourage the expulsion of uric acid from the body.

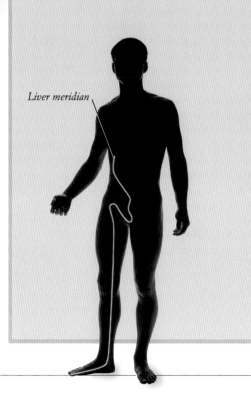

Spleen/ pancreas meridian

Stomach meridian

Liver meridian

LEFT

THE SPLEEN/ PANCREAS MERIDIAN AND THE LIVER MERIDIAN ARE FOUND ON THE BIG TOE. MOST SUFFERERS FROM BUNIONS ALSO HAVE SPLEEN/ PANCREAS DISORDERS. THE STOMACH MERIDIAN RUNS THROUGH THE SECOND TOE, SO HAMMERTOE SUFFERERS OFTEN HAVE STOMACH DISORDERS.

Skin Problems

CALLUSES

Repeated pressure and friction on the skin will cause it to thicken into a callus as a means of protection. Foot calluses are quite common because the skin on the feet is subject to a great deal of pressure, especially from ill-fitting shoes. Calluses grow on flat surfaces and have no nucleus. They most often appear on the weight-bearing part of the foot such as the heel or the ball, as well as on the tops of the toes. Calluses also often form on the cushions of the toes – usually the fourth and fifth toes. These particular calluses have the appearance of a thick, sharp "knife-edge." The big toe, too, is prone to callus formation. Sports, shoes, and long periods of standing may contribute to their development. A callus is usually a sign of uneven weight distribution.

If this thickening is aggravated by consistent pressure, the buildup of skin will lead to pain and discomfort. Burning sensations in the callus or congestion and swelling under it indicate that it is irritating nerve endings. If severe, it may require surgery and is easily removed by a chiropodist. If the reason for it forming is not dealt with, it will inevitably recur.

CORNS

Corns, a common foot complaint, also develop as a means of protection. They are one of the most prevalent disorders of the musculoskeletal system. Corns are cone-shaped, have no root, and usually develop on the joints of toes, because of their relative prominence. Toes are particularly sensitive to pressure from shoes.

At the focal point of pressure, the skin hardens and thickens. A corn – basically a concentrated area of hard skin – forms in the middle of the thickening where the pressure is greatest. Recurrent friction irritates the area, stimulating increased blood supply, which in turn accelerates cell growth. Corns also develop on the soles of the feet in areas that are regularly subject to excessive pressure.

Stabbing pain occurs when the central "eye" descends into the tissue and the hard skin exerts secondary pressure onto the sensitive tissue and nerve endings.

BELOW
Corns have developed here on the tops of deformed hammertoes.

CORNS AND CALLUSES ARE COMMON FOOT COMPLAINTS, USUALLY CAUSED BY CONSTANT PRESSURE OR FRICTION OR BY SEVERE IMBALANCES IN THE SIX MERIDIANS FOUND ON THE FOOT.

ABOVE
A corn is a disk of hard tissue surrounded by reddened skin, in this case on an adult's little toe. The hard tissue forms an inverted pyramid, which presses down into the deeper layers of the skin, causing pain.

MERIDIANS AND SKIN PROBLEMS

Corns and calluses may develop on the heel and ball of the foot, and the tops of the toes. It is important to note exactly where these appear and establish on which meridian and reflex they manifest to establish which organs are out of balance. For example, the stomach meridian runs along the second and third toes, and problems here indicate congestions along the stomach meridian. Symptoms such as acidity, gastritis, ulcers, appendix and tonsil trouble, sinus, skin problems, and breast problems are often found in people with corns and calluses on the second and third toes.

The second toe is also often longer than the first toe. This can indicate a genetic weakness in the stomach, which is often inherited but can also be due to deficiencies of particular nutrients in the mother's diet during pregnancy. This can cause nutritional deficiencies in the developing embryo, which can later manifest as stomach weakness. If the weakness is genetic, care should always be taken with diet, for example, avoiding excessively acid foods.

Some people have a long callus under the second toe. This relates to the bronchi/throat reflex area. If there is a deep groove in the skin it could also relate to a weakness in the throat, and the person may have a tendency to suffer from throat, tonsil, and bronchial problems. The stomach meridian traverses through the throat area – tonsils, thyroid, and the throat itself. The stomach meridian is on top of the second toe, while the throat and bronchi reflexes are on the soles between the first and second toes. Moving down, the meridian runs underneath the bone region – the thyroid. Many people have a groove or hard callus around the bone, which can again be related to an imbalance in the spleen/pancreas and stomach meridians, since these are closely related. Hard skin over the lung reflex is also a common problem. This can indicate a weak chest. The stomach meridian also runs through the lung area and the gall bladder meridian enters the lung area from the side.

As you can see, it is important to take careful note of where corns and calluses form and refer them to the meridians in order to understand the root cause of the problem.

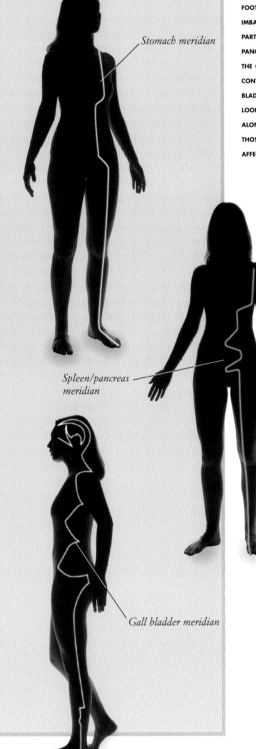

Stomach meridian

Spleen/pancreas meridian

Gall bladder meridian

BELOW

THE STOMACH MERIDIAN RUNS THROUGH THE SECOND AND THIRD TOES, SO CORNS AND CALLUSES THERE MAY ALSO BE ASSOCIATED WITH STOMACH DISORDERS. A CALLUS FURTHER UNDER THE FOOT CAN INDICATE AN IMBALANCE ON THE PARTNER SPLEEN/PANCREAS MERIDIAN. THE OUTER TOES CONTAIN THE GALL BLADDER MERIDIAN, SO LOOK FOR PROBLEMS ALONG THIS MERIDIAN IF THOSE TOES ARE AFFECTED.

ATHLETE'S FOOT

Athlete's foot is a fungal infection that usually manifests on the skin between the toes. This is the most common site of infection since the moist, warm conditions stimulate the fungus to multiply. The fungus thrives on keratin – a protein found in the outer layers of the skin. A major symptom of this condition is itching, if this is accompanied by loose, scaly skin surrounding patches of pink, exposed skin. Twenty species of fungi may be responsible for athlete's foot.

PLANTAR WARTS

FUNGAL INFECTIONS, SUCH AS ATHLETE'S FOOT, AND VIRAL INFECTIONS, SUCH AS WARTS, AFFECT THE TOES AND SOLES OF THE FEET. ECZEMA, ALTHOUGH NOT CONTAGIOUS, IS ANOTHER SKIN PROBLEM COMMONLY AFFECTING THE FEET.

Warts are believed to be caused by a virus. They appear as an elevation of the skin. This protuberance of skin occurs due to an increase in the size of cells of which the skin tissue is composed. Plantar warts occur on the soles of the feet and can cause much discomfort.

RIGHT
This patient has a ten-day old form the fungal infecti athlete's foot.

ABOVE
The sole of the foot is often a site of athlete's foot. This fungal infection is the most common form of ringworm.

LEFT
Plantar warts are also known as verrucas, occurring on the toes and soles of the feet. The infection is usually acquired from contaminated floors in swimming pools and communal showers.

ECZEMA

This is an acute or chronic inflammatory condition of the skin. The eruption appears first as papules, which become moist and finally form scabs. There is great irritation in the affected part and constitutional disturbances may also be present. If the area affected is dry and scaly it is known as dry eczema. Weeping eczema exhibits a serous exudation from the affected area, which precedes drying up.

BELOW
Chronic eczema on and between this patient's toes.

BELOW
A cluster of plantar warts on a patient's big toe.

Circulation
meridian

Bladder
meridian

MERIDIANS AND ATHLETE'S FOOT

Again, it is important to take note of exactly where on the foot the problem is. Athlete's foot will most often manifest between the fourth and fifth toes – the bladder meridian – and can, therefore, be related to the bladder and its meridian. If between the third and fourth toes, it would be related to imbalances on the gall bladder meridian.

MERIDIANS, REFLEXES, AND PLANTAR WARTS

Many people suffer from this affliction and find the warts extremely difficult to eradicate – they often reappear after surgical removal. An elderly client had five warts on his heart reflex that had appeared after major heart surgery. Again, observe where they appear and relate the position to a reflex, meridian, and organ. Reflexology treatment helps strengthen the problem organ, thus correcting the imbalance. As a result, the warts often disappear.

MERIDIANS, REFLEXES, AND ECZEMA

The same principle applies here as in the other example above; relate the area where the problem manifests to reflexes, meridians, and organs to ascertain the extent of the problem area.

LEFT
BY CHECKING CAREFULLY TO SEE ON WHICH MERIDIAN A PROBLEM OCCURS, THE REFLEXOLOGIST CAN LOCATE AREAS OF AFFLICATION IN THE BODY.

Relate the problem eczema area to the relevant meridian.

Toenail Problems

INGROWING TOENAIL

As anyone who suffers from this problem knows, an ingrowing toenail can be extremely painful and uncomfortable. It is interesting to note that those most often affected by this condition are young people in their teens and twenties. It usually occurs on the big toe when the side of the nail penetrates the skin of the nail groove and becomes embedded in the soft skin tissue. If the wound is hampered in its efforts to heal, it produces granulation tissue, which accumulates on the side and top of the nail. The tissue bleeds easily and can become infected. Sometimes a callus forms as a protective measure.

Ingrowing toenails can be caused by cutting the nail too short or cutting down the sides of the nail. The correct way to cut a toenail is straight across. Thin, brittle nails and moist skin will increase susceptibility to this problem.

THICKENED TOENAIL

A toenail will thicken if the nail cell production center is damaged. This can happen if the nail rubs persistently against a shoe over a prolonged period, or if the toenail has sustained injury in an accident. Unfortunately this condition is irreversible. A further complication arises as the nail grows; the new growth curves and is unsightly and uncomfortable. This curvature is known as a "rams-horn" nail. Many elderly people suffer from this.

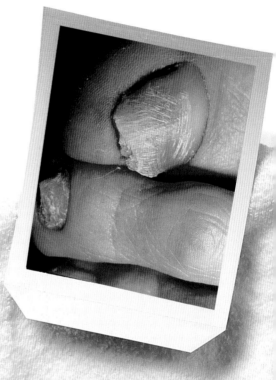

RIGHT
Chronic fungal infection of the toenail can be caused by the dermatophyte fungus, as here, or by problems on the spleen/ pancreas meridian. The patient may have to take drugs for up to a year to ensure that the infection is cleared.

TOENAIL PROBLEMS CAN BE CAUSED BY INFECTION, DAMAGE TO THE NAIL CELL PRODUCTION CENTER, OR CUTTING THE NAIL TOO SHORT.

ABOVE
The toenail on this patient's big toe is ingrowing toward the second toe. The surrounding skin is swollen, bleeding and infected.

INVOLUTED TOENAIL

An involuted toenail, if not correctly tended, can develop into an ingrowing toenail. This condition occurs when the normal curve of the toenail is so exaggerated that it produces pain down the side of the nail. The exaggerated curve can also encourage the development of corns and calluses on the sides of the nail, which will increase discomfort.

It is difficult to cut this type of involuted nail. Cutting down the sides must be avoided, since this will result in the new nail growth forcing its way through the soft skin at the side of the nail eventually causing an ingrowing toenail.

FUNGAL INFECTION OF THE TOENAIL

This condition – also known as ony-chomycosis – often accompanies athlete's foot. The fungus penetrates the nail causing it to thicken. If the condition deteriorates, the color and texture of the nail will also be affected. Warning signs are change of color of the toenail to a chalky or yellowish shade with a distinct odor. The nail edge looks granular and acquires a sandlike texture. It is advisable to seek treatment for this condition quickly.

MERIDIANS AND TOENAIL TROUBLES

With all toenail troubles, it is imperative that meridians are taken into account. Take, for example, ingrowing toenails. This problem is often found in young people and situated on the big toe – the spleen/pancreas meridian. These people usually have a diet high in sugar, junk food, alcohol, and cigarettes, and many of their problems can be related to sugar metabolism or pancreatic disorder. The big toe is also the head reflex, and people with ingrowing toenails often tend to suffer from headaches and migraines.

Check the section on meridians and note which ones run through the area of the foot where the physical deformities and problems are found to ascertain which organ is congested and needs correcting.

LEFT
The inflammation of this patient's second toe is due to cellulitis, a bacterial infection of the connective tissue below the skin.

Spleen/pancreas meridian

...nychia, a ...rial ...tion caused ...or foot ...ne, has ...ted this ... big toe.

LEFT
AN INGROWING TOENAIL ON THE BIG TOE CAN INDICATE PROBLEMS ON THE SPLEEN/PANCREAS MERIDIANS.

109

Toes and Arches

FLAT FEET (PES PLANUS)

Flat feet can be caused by numerous factors. They are often inherited but may also develop due to weakness in the joints, "overloading" the feet, or as a result of a long illness. In childhood this condition can occur if growth is too rapid or if the child is malnourished or overweight. The weaker the foot, the greater the possibility that this condition will develop in consequence.

If not inherited, flat feet can be identified if the ankles lean toward each other. This means that the joint beneath the ankle is out of order, resulting in a weak ankle. Or the ligaments of the foot may literally collapse because of walking injuries or incorrect walking habits. The ligaments may lose control and the foot will spread to become square-shaped.

Hallmarks of a fallen arch are fatigue and pain, ranging from a sore arch to aches up to the knee. In addition to causing an unattractive style of walking, flat feet can also affect the spine. The spine becomes more vulnerable as the foot no longer acts as an efficient shock absorber and thus impacts reverberate upward with more force.

Too much standing weakens the ligaments responsible for holding the foot in one piece. As these give way the longitudinal heel-to-toe arch lowers with them; stress registers in the lower back. Back pain is a common sign of this kind of foot trouble. Foot pain or "burning" soles could indicate strain on the longitudinal arches. Specific exercises may be used to build up muscle strength. Commercial arch supports are available.

Overstretching and weakness of both muscles and tendons place a strain on the bone structure. Another problem is that nerves and blood vessels, usually protected from contact with the ground by the shape of the arch, are now subject to pressure and their condition will deteriorate, affecting the reflexes in this area.

BELOW
In flat feet the sole lies flat on the ground. The condition can be caused by prolonged standing, as well as being due to overweight or inheritance.

— Aching legs

— Ankle leans inward

— Sole lies flat on ground

Weak joint

Pressure on nerves and blood vessels

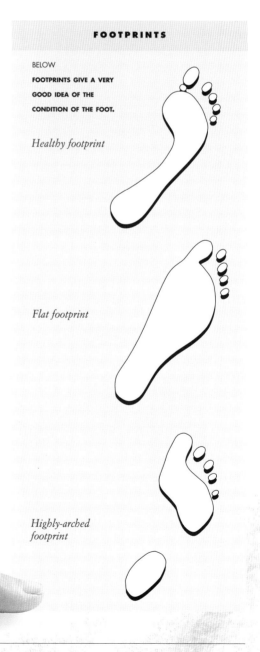

FOOTPRINTS

BELOW

FOOTPRINTS GIVE A VERY GOOD IDEA OF THE CONDITION OF THE FOOT.

Healthy footprint

Flat footprint

Highly-arched footprint

THE HIGHLY ARCHED FOOT
(PES CAVUS)

The highly arched foot is usually stiff, which limits maneuverability and prevents efficient functioning of the foot. This condition tends to be transmitted genetically and often only requires well-fitted shoes or metatarsal arch supports to correct the weight-bearing pattern. The head of the metatarsals may ache because of the shape of the foot, and calluses may develop since so much pressure is exerted on the toes and ball of the foot.

Because of the exaggerated height of the arch, the toes will not have correct contact with the ground when standing. The unnatural shape and position of the toes – they are curled under in a configuration known as a "clawfoot" – makes them particularly susceptible to external pressures and prone to corns and calluses.

In addition to the possibility of hereditary influences, this condition could also be the result of nerve and muscle imbalance. It is often witnessed in the neurological conditions poliomyelitis and spina bifida. These arch problems usually require surgical correction.

THE ARCH AND REFLEXOLOGY

As a reflexologist I perceive the problem of flat feet as being a rigid spine, indicating that the person is not supple and could also be inclined to lower back problems. A highly curved arch or curved spine reflex also indicates a spinal problem, and this can affect the upper part of the body in the chest (thoracic) area.

If you press your fist against the lung reflex on the foot and gently push the foot back into the normal position, you will see the spine "correcting" itself. Any problems relating to the spine reflex indicate that the person may have a tendency to lower back problems, neck tension, and congestions in the lung area. As the toes are also often affected, there will be problems related to the meridians in the toes.

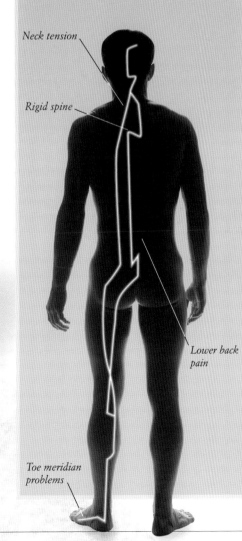

Neck tension

Rigid spine

Lower back pain

Toe meridian problems

FAR LEFT
Clawfoot can be helped by using a molded insole in the shoe to redistribute body weight evenly over the foot. Extreme cases may require surgery to cut a tendon on the underside of the foot and flatten the foot out.

LEFT
THE SPINE REFLEXES APPEAR ON THE ARCH OF THE FOOT. PROBLEMS HERE WILL BE REFLECTED ALONG THE CLIENT'S BACK IN THE FORM OF LOWER BACK PAIN OR NECK TENSION.

LEFT
Problems along the gall bladder meridian manifest themselves on the fourth toe, which here shows signs of a tendency to swelling.

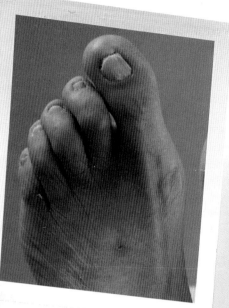

RIGHT
Any toe may become enlarged. An enlarged big toe, as here, indicates problems on the spleen/ pancreas meridian.

RIGHT
HIP PROBLEMS ARE OFTEN ASSOCIATED WITH THE GALL BLADDER MERIDIAN, WHICH CAN BE REFLECTED ON THE CUBOID BONE.

Gall bladder meridian

THE HEEL IS SUBJECT TO AN INTENSE AMOUNT OF PRESSURE, WHICH CAN RESULT IN FISSURES OR SPURS.

PLANTAR DIGITAL NEURITIS

Neuritis is the inflammation of a nerve causing pain, tenderness, and loss of function. This particular form of neuritis affects the toes, specifically the fourth toe. The pain begins at the web between the third and fourth toes and shoots up into the fourth toe. The sensations experienced in the toe may vary from slight numbness to intense pain, depending on how severely the nerve is affected. This discomfort can be alleviated by massaging the toe. This usually occurs in women rather than men.

ENLARGED TOES

Sometimes the cushions of the toes become so enlarged they seem deformed. This can occur on any toe but often manifests on the fourth toe – the gall bladder meridian – again indicating imbalances along the meridian or the reflex.

URETER/BLADDER WEAKNESS

The ureter reflex runs across the arch on the sole of the foot, extending from the kidney reflex to the bladder reflex. This can be visible as a clear "line" in the skin, and indicates a history of kidney/bladder disorders or weakness. The bladder reflex may clearly appear as a puffy area, again indicating weakness.

BELOW
The bladder reflex appears as a puffy area, indicating weakness.

MERIDIANS AND PLANTAR DIGITAL NEURITIS

The gall bladder meridian is found on the fourth toe, where a plantar digital neuritis problem is most common. It occurs in many women, and I have witnessed numerous cases where women have this problem around premenstrual time when they often crave chocolates, caffeine, and other stimulants that overload the gall bladder. Often, symptoms will indicate other problems that are related to the gall bladder.

It can also be associated with hip trouble and can possibly be seen as a puffy area in line with the fourth toe close to the ankle. The gall bladder meridian runs through the hip region, and swelling here may indicate congestion along the gall bladder meridian. In some cases this may manifest as a posture problem that stems from the hip region.

The Heel

The heel is subject to immense stress – it bears the brunt of walking and a great deal of body weight. The heel bone is the largest bone in the foot. Walking takes its toll on this bone, so it has a protective thick layer of fatty tissue.

HEEL CALLUS

This is formed when areas of skin around the edge of the heel become thicker than usual to protect it from aggravating pressure and friction. It can develop into a painful condition if not dealt with.

HEEL FISSURE

A heel fissure develops when the skin on the edge of the heel splits – usually due to the fact that the skin is excessively dry and is being pinched in ill-fitting shoes. If the fissure is deep, pain and bleeding can occur, and it may also become infected.

HEEL SPUR

This is a bony growth on the underside of the heel bone. Overweight people develop spurs due to excess weight bearing down on the heels. Spurs are the result of a torn longitudinal ligament that bleeds and generates fibrous tissue that ultimately calcifies. It is sometimes accompanied by pain and inflammation.

RIGHT
This heel callus is caused by excessive pressure exerted on the patient's foot as a result of a polio deformity.

LEFT
This patient's ill-fitting shoes caused this heel spur.

RIGHT
These jogger's heels are badly inflamed with heel spurs and heel calluses on both feet – the result of pressure from running shoes.

BELOW
PROBLEMS ON THE HEEL ARE OFTEN REFLECTED IN THE CORRESPONDING PELVIC AREA OF THE BODY.

MERIDIANS, REFLEXES, AND HEEL PROBLEMS

The heel is the pelvic reflex and imbalances here will often indicate prostate problems in men and uterus problems in women. Many women have deep cracks in their heels just prior to a hysterectomy and these often heal naturally after the operation. Other reproductive problems in men and women – infertility, heavy menstrual bleeding and discomfort – can be related to imbalances in the pelvic region. All six main meridians run through this area, and organs and meridians can be stimulated by massage of the heel area.

Another fissure may occur at the anus/rectum reflex below the inner ankle bone, where the heel meets the arch. This can be related to tendencies to hemorrhoids or a spastic colon.

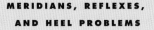

Deep cracks in heel

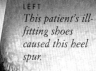

Prostate problems

Hemorrhoids and spastic colon problems

Fissure at anus/ rectum reflex

Case Study 1

What can a reflexologist learn from your feet? He or she can combine observations of the feet with a knowledge of the meridian pathways and characteristics to produce an accurate picture of a client's state of health.

PATIENT: 25-YEAR-OLD FEMALE

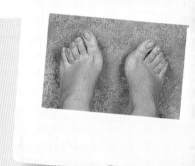

THE BIG TOES

Both sides of the big toes lean toward the other toes showing the start of bunions and also calluses. The area of the bunion corresponds to the thyroid reflex.

In looking at bunions an "emotional thyroid" can often be seen – a person in need of stimulants and often feeling close to tears. The liver meridian is found on the "inside" of the big toenail and the spleen/pancreas on the "outside" of the nail. If the spleen is in disharmony, the whole body or some part of it may develop deficient ch'i or deficient blood.

SPLEEN/PANCREAS MERIDIAN CONGESTIONS

- Irregular menstrual cycle.
- Painful shins, especially when taking stimulants, such as tea with sugar.
- Recent weight gain of 30lb. (earth element), energy levels low, experiences stress at work.
- Lumps removed from outside of left breast; two Caesarean sections.
- Lips dry and sore and cracked in the corners (relating to the earth element).

Spleen/pancreas meridian

Element symbols
Each meridian is linked to an element (see pages 64–83), the characteristics of which can be reflected in a patient's state of health.

THE SECOND AND THIRD TOES

We see that there are corns on the tops of the second and third toes, which relate to the stomach meridian.

The stomach controls digestion – it receives nourishment, integrates it and passes on the "pure" food energy to be distributed by the partner, spleen.

Stom[ach] mer[idian]

STOMACH MERIDIAN CONGESTIONS

- Sinus, postnasal drip, and allergies: eczema on sides of nose.
- Wisdom teeth removed. Teeth have fillings.
- Eyes itchy from allergies.
- Blue shadows under eyes – indicating excessive stress placed on kidneys.
- Complexion flushed and red. Here, the client has a tight chest and shortness of breath and suffers from recurring laryngitis.
- Tonsils and appendix removed at an early age.
- Suffers from hiatus hernia and ovarian pain.
- Skin blemishes on left thigh directly on stomach meridian.

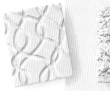

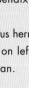

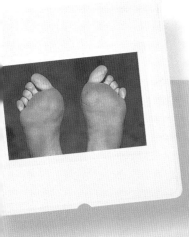

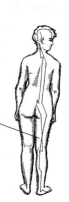

Bladder meridian

THE FIFTH TOES

There is a corn on the top of the little toes (bladder meridian) and knife-shaped calluses underneath the little toes (kidney meridian). The bladder reflex is puffy. She experiences pain along her Achilles tendon (on kidney meridian.)

BLADDER MERIDIAN CONGESTIONS
- Cramping calves and corns on little toes.
- Varicose veins on bladder meridian.
- Bladder works overtime at night.

Wood element characteristics
- *Like of food flavored excessively with sour ingredients (flavor).*
- *Responds best regarding her health to spring (season).*
- *Weak ligaments and tendons in feet (tissues).*
- *Eyes becoming weaker (sense organ).*
- *Tends toward aggressiveness for no apparent reason (emotion).*

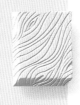

THE FOURTH TOES

The fourth toe shows a corn on the top of her right foot and a corn on the side of the fourth toe on the left foot, which is rubbing against the little toe and the toe is being "pulled" out of line. The fourth toe relates to the gall bladder meridian.

The liver/gall bladder is responsible for the integrity of the ligaments and tendons.

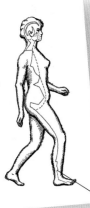

Gall bladder meridian

Water element characteristics
- *Weak teeth (tissues).*
- *Dislike of cold weather (climate) and winter (season).*
- *Head hair dry and brittle (tissues).*
- *Phobia of confined spaces (emotion).*
- *Nails are soft and peel easily (tissues).*

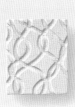

FURTHER FEATURES TO NOTE
Both cuboids protrude indicating a weakness in the hip region relating to the reflexes. The gall bladder meridian runs through the hip and also runs through part of the hip reflex on the sides of the feet. The client suffers from shooting pains beginning in the hips and continuing down the front of her body.

On the partner meridian, the liver, we find that the client suffers from recurring vaginal thrush (candida albicans).

Case Study 2

This case study demonstrates how the accumulative, progressive state of disease is reflected in the structural abnormalities of the client's feet. As the parent of the client in the previous case study, this client's feet also reflect the potential pathway of her daughter's health, should her daughter choose not to change her lifestyle and thereby halt the further deterioration of her body.

PATIENT: 67-YEAR-OLD FEMALE

This patient is the mother of the client in the case study on pages 114–115.

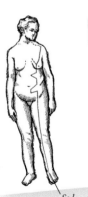

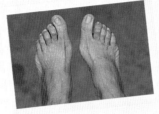

THE SECOND AND THIRD TOES

The partner meridian to the spleen/pancreas, the stomach meridian, appears on the second and third toes. Here the client has hammertoes and also has corns on the tops of the second toes.

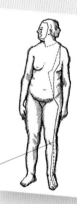

Stomach meridian

THE BIG TOES

Both big toes, on which the spleen/pancreas meridian appears, lean toward all the other toes, creating bunions. This indicates an emotional pancreas affecting the thyroid and reflecting the need to hide behind stimulants. Her thyroid reflex has a callus and she is taking thyroid medication.

Spleen/ pancreas meridian

SPLEEN/PANCREAS MERIDIAN CONGESTIONS

- Lumps removed from the outside of both breasts.
- Menstruation was heavy and irregular when the client was young and she underwent a hysterectomy.

STOMACH MERIDIAN CONGESTIONS

- Suffers from sinus and postnasal drip, and like her daughter, has shadows under the eyes showing a weakness in the kidneys due to digestive problems.
- False teeth. Her daughter also shows progressive weakness in this area.
- Evidence on her cheek of problems in the bronchi region. Cheeks have broken capillaries. Frequently suffers from chest congestion and is a heavy smoker.
- She also has a strong callus on the esophagus reflex and sometimes has flatulence and heartburn.

Earth element characteristics
- *Strong desire for tea and cigarettes (flavor).*
- *Excessive need for love and attention (emotion).*

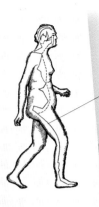

Gall bladder meridian

Kidney meridian

THE FOURTH TOES

Her gall bladder meridian shows congestion in the form of knee pain on the left lateral side of the knee. She also has varicose veins along the meridian on her legs. Her cuboid bones also protrude (as found in her daughter) and reflect problems in the hip region.

GALL BLADDER MERIDIAN CONGESTIONS

- Hip pain and difficulty in bending.
- Difficulty in digesting fatty foods and becomes nauseous.
- Varicose veins on the gall bladder meridian.
- Knee pain on lateral side.

THE FIFTH TOES

Observing the little toes, we find a callus underneath toward the shoulder reflex. She suffers from shoulder pain along the top of the meridian. There are corns on the tops of her little toes. She also suffers from burning soles – mainly along the kidney meridian in the instep.

BLADDER MERIDIAN CONGESTIONS

- Suffers from headaches along the bladder meridian across the crown.
- Shoulder pain.
- Had a prolapsed bladder and urination is slow.
- Corns on tops of little toes.

Wood element characteristics
- *Weak eyes (sense organ).*
- *Healthier in the spring (season).*
- *Dislikes the color green (color).*
- *Dislikes sour flavors (flavor).*
- *Emotions tend toward aggressiveness (emotion).*

Water element characteristics
- *Energy poor – especially in the late afternoon (3p.m. – 7p.m.).*
- *Ill every winter (season).*
- *Dislikes the cold (climate).*
- *Loves the color blue (color).*
- *Fear of using elevators (emotion).*
- *Has a groaning sound in voice (sound).*
- *Nails are brittle – so were teeth (now has false). Hair dry and brittle (tissues).*

Case Study 3

This case history further illustrates the genetically inherited weaknesses reflected in the case studies on pages 114–117. Several signs on the feet are practically identical between the members of the family. Furthermore, the actual complaints that manifest along the common meridians are also similar.

PATIENT: 28-YEAR-OLD MALE

This patient is the son of the client in the case study on pages 116–117.

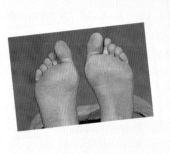

THE SECOND AND THIRD TOES

The partner meridian, the stomach meridian, is found on the second and third toes. Here the toes show dorsal lifting on both sides, far more so than on the other toes; these could develop into hammertoes like those of his mother. Plantar warts on the lung reflex under the left foot and calluses on both reflexes confirm weaknesses in the respiratory system.

Gall bladder meridian

Cuboid bone

Stomach meridian

THE BIG TOES

Both big toes, through which the spleen/pancreas meridian runs, lean toward all the other toes showing the potential to create bunions. This is indicative of disharmony in the pancreas, particularly emotionally, affecting the thyroid and reflecting the need to hide behind stimulants. His thyroid reflex has a callus.

Earth element characteristics

- *Strong desire for tea and cigarettes (flavor).*
- *Excessive need for love and attention (emotion).*
- *Damp climate constricts his chest (climate).*
- *Drools onto his pillow while sleeping (fluid secretion).*

STOMACH MERIDIAN CONGESTIONS

- Suffers from sinus problems like his mother and sister, also evidence on his cheeks of problems in the bronchi region (broken capillaries in common with his mother).
- Suffers from a "feeling of lack of oxygen" when subjected to stress and has a corresponding tightness in the chest. Experiences a scratchy irritation in the throat. Snores, and breathing is worse at night. Has had bronchitis and other lung congestions.
- Blue shadows underneath the eyes indicative of stress on the urinary system, again, like his sister, due to an imbalance with the stomach meridian. Has had a peptic ulcer. Often suffers from flatulence and heartburn – like his mother.
- Has had his tonsils and appendix removed – like his sister.
- Underwent surgery to small intestine due to problems at birth.
- Has had a hernia problem – like his sister.
- Frequently has problems with bowel movements, constipation and diarrhea.

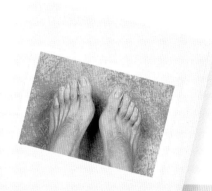

Wood element characteristics

- *Weak eyes (sense organ).*
- *Eyes often watery (fluid secretion).*
- *Health best in the spring (season).*
- *Emotions tend toward aggressiveness (emotion).*

Kidney meridian

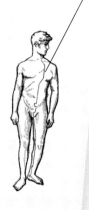

THE FOURTH TOES

Moving on to the fourth toe and the gall bladder meridian and its partner, the liver meridian, which is found in the big toe, we find that like his mother and sister, all his toes lift up dorsally showing weakness in the ligaments and tendons. On his feet he shows signs that confirm his liver weakness and these appear as calluses in the liver reflex.

lder
ridian

GALL BLADDER MERIDIAN CONGESTIONS

- He suffers from occasional back problems and stiffness in the hip region.
- Headaches lateral to the eye.
- Toes lift dorsally.
- Weak tendons and ligaments.

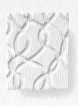

Water element characteristics

- *Bad quality head hair (physical manifestations).*
- *Favorite color is blue (color).*
- *Dislikes cold climate (climate).*
- *Phobia of heights (emotion).*
- *Nails soft and peeling (tissues).*
- *Bouts of deafness (sense organ).*

THE FIFTH TOES

The two meridians on both sides of the fifth toes, the bladder and kidney meridians, show a knife-shaped callus, and the toenails are hard and fungal. His bladder reflex is puffy and there are lines running from the kidney to the bladder reflex, indicating a weakness in that region. This is confirmed by the fact that he has problems urinating – flow is sluggish. There is a fissure at the anus/rectum reflex on his feet.

BLADDER MERIDIAN CONGESTIONS

- Going bald.
- He suffers from lower back pain and often has painful hemorrhoids.
- Fungal toenail on little toe.

FURTHER FEATURES TO NOTE

Like his mother and sister, most of his congestions are manifest along the meridians found in the feet, with a few exceptions. On the small intestine, he suffers from tinnitus. The little fingers on his hands are irregularly short – the little finger relating to the small intestine and its partner, the heart meridian (a weakness here already having made itself manifest at birth). The plantar wart on his left foot is perhaps indicative of future problems with his heart. He already experiences palpitations. His blood vessels (tissues) are weak. He has varicose veins and his feet are always cold. On an emotional level, he alternates between a lack of enthusiasm for life and a state of hyperexcitability.

10. WHAT IS A REFLEXOLOGY TREATMENT LIKE?

A reflexology treatment should be an extremely pleasurable experience. Many people may feel somewhat apprehensive at the prospect of their first reflexology treatment, so it is the reflexologist's responsibility to ensure that the client is made to feel welcome and comfortable. Practitioners should try to be caring and compassionate and reassure clients that they are "in good hands." Since relaxation is of prime importance in the healing process, the surroundings must be as peaceful and organized as possible. Once the session has begun, all distractions must be avoided. Telephone interruptions or children and dogs rushing in and out will not assist in achieving the desired effect!

BELOW
A relaxed environment with no distractions enables the reflexologist to concentrate on the client and helps to promote a feeling of well-being in the client.

Couch

Detailed case history

Some people have strange attitudes regarding their feet and many will be embarrassed about the state of their feet. Any insecurities of this type must be dispelled. Feet are a reflexologist's domain – they specialize in feet and are accustomed to seeing them in all shapes, sizes, and conditions. The feet represent the body and encompass a wealth of information about one's state of health. They are the key to revealing where imbalances lie and play a vital role in the enhancement of general health and well-being.

MEDICAL HISTORY

At the first treatment, the practitioner begins by taking a thorough medical history. All problems must be noted, not just those troubling the client at the time. This level of detail is necessary because all problems are relevant in ascertaining a complete health picture.

In order to understand the client and his or her complaint, it is advisable to record a detailed case history. This is useful to refer back to during ensuing treatments to gage progress. The example of a case history sheet (page 121) can serve as a guideline, but obviously individual

Oil   Herbal cream   Soft, freshly laundered towels   Plaster model of foot

PATIENT RECORD

Name AMELIA WRIGHT

Address 15 Montrose Street, Eastergate, Chichester West Sussex PO21 7RU **Telephone** 01432 454347

Complaint Headaches - forehead, neck tension (bladder), tendency to bladder infections, lower back pain, sinus, feels nauseous when eating rich food (gall bladder), pain around outer breast with menstrual cycle, vaginal infections (candida)

Treatments tried:

Medication Painkiller

Blood pressure Normal

Bowels Constipation

Headaches Forehead/neck

Energy Feels tired most of the time

Mind "slightly" forgetful

Stress Has lots of stress at work

Digestion Heartburn often

Exercise None

Vitamin supplements None

Tongue slightly split

Skin/Hair/Nails White spots on index finger (colon)

Endocrine Irregular, heavy & painful menstrual cycle, PMS

Operations Tonsils, appendix

Sleep Erratic

Meridians Bladder (headaches, eyes, and lower back), stomach (sinus, gall bladder, colon), spleen, pancreas (vaginal and breast)

Eyes Wears glasses

Weight +- 58 kg

Diet Breakfast = cereal & fruits
Lunch = bread, cheese, tomato
Supper = meat, vegetables
Liquids = 6-8 cups of tea and fruit juice. Often wine with dinner.

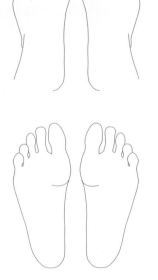

Treatment results

2nd After 1st treatment, headache was worse for 2 days, felt v. tired;
3rd Headaches a lot less & less painful, still lower back;
4th Menstrual cycle was easier, less pain, only slight PMS, colon fine;
5th Bowels moving every day, had no headaches, candida a lot better;
6th Has had no heartburn - feels good.

LEFT
A detailed record of the client's complaint, personal details, and treatment should be kept for future reference.

practitioners will develop their own to suit their specific requirements. The following offers a "practitioner's eye view" on compiling a case history.

First note the complaint for which treatment is being sought. Then take note of all other symptoms and operations in as much detail as possible. If headaches occur on· the bladder meridian, check whether the client has a history of bladder problems. If they occur on the gall bladder meridian, other symptoms may include nausea or intolerance of fatty foods, and thus a gall bladder imbalance may be pinpointed as the cause.

CHECKING BODY SYSTEMS

Check thoroughly through each body system, questioning the functions – digestion, bowels, bladder, and blood pressure. Does the client feel mentally alert? How does he or she cope with stress? Is the client's energy level depleted? Does he or she suffer from heartburn or other digestive disorders? What exercise does the client take? Observe the skin, hair, and nail condition and record this. Check the tongue, since this provides an insight into the condition of the stomach. A clean tongue usually indicates that the digestive system is functioning normally, while a tongue with a white or yellow coating could indicate a congestion or imbalance in the digestive system.

What of the endocrine system? If female, record all problems related to the menstruation and premenstrual tension symptoms. Also record all previous operations. In this way one can determine which meridian dominates the problems.

Question how the problem developed, how long it has been present, accompanying aches and pains, eating and drinking habits, parents' eating habits, and hereditary tendencies. For example, you may be treating a mother who may suffer breast problems and painful ovaries, while her child suffers from acne and chest weakness – all symptoms that manifest along the stomach meridian. Hereditary dietary indiscretions can often be cited as the main culprit of the conditions.

It is not wise to force dietary change on a client, but one should try to encourage a more healthy way of eating. Using the stomach meridian as an example, point out problems that can arise from dietary indiscretions. Once the client understands the cause of pain and discomfort, he or she will be more willing to adapt and adopt a different lifestyle.

Keep a comprehensive record of each treatment, checking all reactions, both good and bad, as well as changes in general health. The pair of feet in the bottom right-hand corner of the case history example on page 121 can be useful for recording information. Mark where the problems occur on the feet for easy reference to the relevant meridians.

REFLEXOLOGISTS DON'T

Reflexologists don't practice medicine. That is the realm of orthodox licenced physicians.

Reflexologists never diagnose diseases, prescribe or adjust medication.

They do not treat specific diseases although reflexology helps eliminate problems caused by specific diseases. By bringing the body back into a state of balance, reflexology treatment can combat a number of disorders. Tender reflexes indicate which parts of the body are congested. This "diagnosis" is only of parts of the body "out of balance," not specific named disorders. It is important to be aware of this. Any attempt to diagnose or prescribe could land a well-meaning reflexologist in a law court.

The Treatment

Once all the relevant details are noted, the treatment can proceed. The receiver must be seated comfortably, preferably on a soft treatment couch with the head and neck well supported, so that you have eye contact. The lower legs should be well supported with the feet in a comfortable position. Shoes, socks, pantyhose, or stockings must be removed and tight garments should be loosened so as not to hinder circulation.

The reflexologist begins by bathing the feet with absorbent cotton soaked in disinfectant. Alternatively, he or she may use a foot spa to which a mild disinfectant is added. Both the feet should be completely dry prior to commencing treatment. The first physical contact is then a gentle stroking movement; then comes a general examination of the feet. Every individual is different, as are their feet.

Temperature, static buildup, muscle tone, tissue tone, and skin condition, as well as deformities, provide a comprehensive picture of the client's problems.

Cold, bluish, or reddish feet indicate poor circulation. Sweaty feet indicate hormonal imbalance. Dry skin could indicate poor circulation. Swelling and puffiness, especially around the ankles, can be related to a variety of internal problems. Tense feet indicate tension in the body, and limp feet indicate poor muscle tone. Foot deformities are also revealing and are discussed in detail in the chapter on "Interpreting the Feet." Special care must be taken with infectious areas since they could spread to other areas of the foot, and to you. Infectious areas should be covered with a bandage or absorbent cotton before being carefully worked on. Avoid working on areas of the feet and ankles where varicose veins are present since this could further damage the veins.

Reflexologists commence with a full treatment as described in "The Treatment Sequence in Detail." Working through all the reflexes activates the organs and body systems and enables reflexologists to determine sore reflex points that indicate areas of congestion. Eye contact is important. Most clients will react in some way – usually loudly – when a sore point is located. Some, however, are stubborn and refuse to react. With eye contact, you will be able to ascertain when a sensitive area is located.

ABOVE
Before treatment begins the reflexologist bathes the client's feet with disinfectant.

ABOVE
A gentle stroking movement relieves tension in the client's feet and relaxes the body.

RIGHT
To reassure the client the reflexologist will describe the treatment before working on the feet.

Couch

Relaxed, happy client

Client's case history

Feet ready for treatment

Soft, clean towel

The treatment must always be gentle but firm. The receiver should never feel that his or her foot is in a vicelike grip and cannot be withdrawn. This could cause tension from the fear that treatment might be painful. The pressure should never be more than is comfortable, but should be sufficiently firm to activate the body's healing potential.

SENSATIONS

Sensations vary on different parts of the feet depending on the functioning of the related body part. Congested areas will be sensitive – the more sensitive, the more congested. The sensations range from the feeling of something sharp (like a piece of glass) being pressed into the foot, to a dull ache, discomfort, tightness, or just firm pressure. Sensitivity varies from person to person. This also varies from treatment to treatment, depending on factors such as stress, mood, and time of day. In many cases, a client may feel little or no tenderness at all during the first treatment. This does not necessarily mean that no areas are congested. More often than not, it indicates an energy blockage in the feet that needs to be freed. The feet usually become more sensitive with subsequent treatments.

As treatment progresses, tenderness should diminish, indicating that balance in a problem area has been restored. The treatment should never be painful or cause the client any discomfort; pressure must be adjusted to suit the individual concerned. Continuous pressure on one point, which could be painful, should be avoided.

Only in the case of an acute pain should tight, continuous pressure be applied to the area that corresponds to the pain – for example, in cases of headache, sciatica, and the like. In these instances apply light pressure for about 15 to 20 seconds on the corresponding reflex. Increase the pressure until the client is just able to tolerate the pain in the reflex area. In most cases acute pain will disappear within a few minutes.

When executing a full treatment, it is important to complete one body part totally before moving on. Both feet are treated alternately in a smooth, even way, since one foot represents half the body. It is, therefore, incorrect to massage one foot completely before moving on to the next foot.

No matter what the sensations, reflexology is always effective and should leave the person feeling light, tingly, and very pampered.

BELOW
The essentials of the treatment room aid the massage techniques and also make the client feel pampered.

Talcum powder absorbs moisture.

Cream keeps skin supple.

Herbal crea healing prop

Clean, soft towels are important for hygiene during treatment.

Soft, clean towels

Reactions to Reflexology Treatment

People differ, so do reactions – and a recipient must be informed of the possible reactions following treatment. On the whole, reactions immediately after a reflexology treatment are largely pleasant, leaving the client feeling calm and relaxed or energized and rejuvenated. However, there is some bad with the good. Reflexology activates the body's own healing power, so some form of reaction is inevitable as the body rids itself of toxins. This is referred to as a "healing crisis" and is a cleansing process. The severity of reactions depends on the degree of imbalance, but should never be too radical. The most common phrase following a first treatment is, "I have never slept so well!"

Most common reactions are related to the body cleansing itself of toxins, as they manifest in the eliminating systems of the body – the kidneys, bowels, skin, and lungs. The following reactions are not generally unusual:

- *Increased urination as the kidneys are stimulated to produce more urine, which may be darker and stronger-smelling due to the toxic content.*
- *Flatulence and more frequent bowel movements.*
- *Aggravated skin condition, particularly in conditions that have been suppressed; increased perspiration; and pimples.*
- *Improved skin tone and tissue texture due to improved circulation.*
- *Increased secretions of the mucous membranes in the nose, mouth, and bronchials.*
- *Disrupted sleep patterns – either deeper or more disturbed sleep.*
- *Dizziness or nausea.*
- *A temporary outbreak of a disease that has been suppressed.*
- *Increased discharge from the vagina in women.*
- *Feverishness.*
- *Tiredness.*
- *Headaches.*
- *Depression, overwhelming desire to weep.*

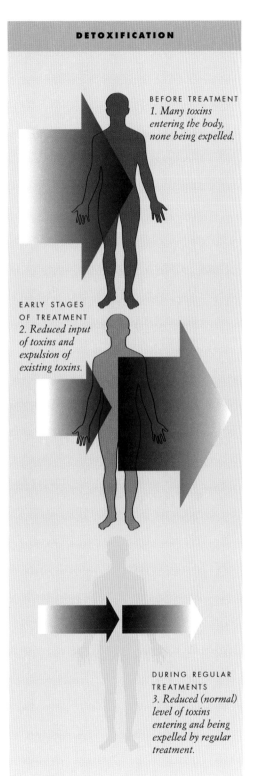

DETOXIFICATION

BEFORE TREATMENT
1. Many toxins entering the body, none being expelled.

EARLY STAGES OF TREATMENT
2. Reduced input of toxins and expulsion of existing toxins.

DURING REGULAR TREATMENTS
3. Reduced (normal) level of toxins entering and being expelled by regular treatment.

LEFT
THE BODY'S HEALING POWER IS ACTIVATED BY REFLEXOLOGY MASSAGE. THE RESULTING "HEALING CRISIS" CLEANSES THE BODY, EXPELLING EXCESS TOXINS AND REGULATING FUTURE INTAKE AND EXPULSION OF TOXINS.

Whatever the reactions, they are a necessary part of the healing process and will pass. Drinking water – preferably warm, boiled water – in place of other liquids will assist in rapidly flushing the toxins from the system.

The Length of a Treatment

The length of the treatment and number of sessions will vary according to the client and the condition. The client's constitution, history and nature of illness, age, body's ability to react to treatment, way of life, and attitude have a profound effect on the healing process. Thus, the degree to which the client responds depends as much on herself or himself as on the practitioner and treatment.

The first treatment session should take approximately one hour. This is the investigative and exploratory stage that enables you to establish as much as possible about the client. Following treatments would last approximately 30 to 50 minutes, depending on the treatment required. If the session is too short, insufficient stimulus is provided for the body to mobilize its own healing powers; if it is too long, there is a danger of overstimulating, which can cause excessive elimination and, therefore, discomfort.

NOTICING IMPROVEMENT

An effect is often experienced immediately after the first treatment. Generally, results are apparent after three or four treatments – either complete or considerable improvement. Well-established disorders will obviously take longer to eradicate than those present for a short time. A course of treatments is recommended for all conditions – even if one session appears to have corrected the problem – to balance the body totally and prevent a recurrence of the disorder. The course should be 8 to 12 treatments once or twice a week. For optimum results, two sessions a week are recommended until there is an improvement, then slowly reduce the frequency. A single treatment won't correct problems that have been developing over several years.

If there is no reaction after several sessions, the body could be unreceptive because of external factors, such as heavy medication or psychological attitude, blocking therapeutic impulses. As long as reactions are positive, there is value in continuing the treatment.

RIGHT
The graph line charts the effectiveness of different treatment durations. The most effective session is about 50 minutes.

0   25 minutes   50 minutes   75 minutes

Too short   Optimum   Too long

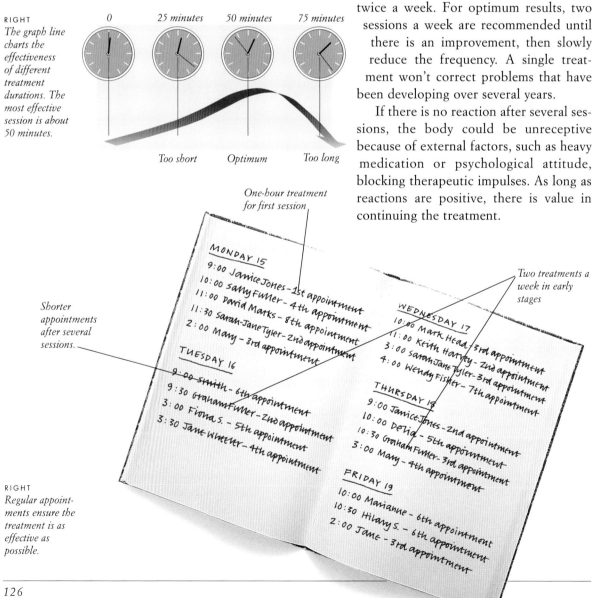

One-hour treatment for first session

Two treatments a week in early stages

Shorter appointments after several sessions.

MONDAY 15
9:00 Janice Jones – 1st appointment
10:00 Sally Fuller – 4th appointment
11:00 David Marks – 8th appointment
11:30 Sarah-Jane Tyler – 2nd appointment
2:00 Mary – 3rd appointment

TUESDAY 16
9:00 Smith – 6th appointment
9:30 Graham Fuller – 2nd appointment
3:00 Fiona S. – 5th appointment
3:30 Jane Wheeler – 4th appointment

WEDNESDAY 17
10:00 Mark Head – 3rd appointment
11:00 Keith Harty – 2nd appointment
3:00 Sarah-Jane Tyler – 3rd appointment
4:00 Wendy Fisher – 7th appointment

THURSDAY 18
9:00 Janice Jones – 2nd appointment
10:00 Delia – 5th appointment
10:30 Graham Fuller – 3rd appointment
3:00 Mary – 4th appointment

FRIDAY 19
10:00 Marianne – 6th appointment
10:30 Hilary S. – 6th appointment
2:00 Jane – 3rd appointment

RIGHT
Regular appointments ensure the treatment is as effective as possible.

The Responsibilities of a Reflexologist

The most important asset a proficient reflexologist can have is genuine compassion for the suffering of humanity and a desire to assist in relieving this suffering. But if you intend to become a practicing reflexologist, you must approach your task with complete and utter professionalism. A thorough knowledge of the subject – reflexes, meridians, foot structure, as well as good basic knowledge of anatomy and physiology – will increase your competence.

A clean, hygienic work space or clinic is necessary to create the correct impression. Grubby, noisy surroundings are hardly the environment in which people seeking health care would wish to find themselves. Everything about the reflexologist should give the impression of professionalism – the surroundings, attire, and approach. To quote from the *Nei Ching*, a profound work widely referred to as the bible of Chinese Medicine: "Poor medical workmanship is neglectful and careless and must, therefore, be combated, because a disease that is not completely cured can easily breed new diseases ... The most important requirement of the art of healing is that no mistakes or neglect occur."[1]

REFLEXOLOGISTS ARE

Professional
Sympathetic to the client
Organized and work in a clean, clinical environment.

Reflexologist explains anatomy of foot.

Patient confident about treatment.

ABOVE
Understanding the anatomy of the foot will help the client to appreciate how reflexology will be beneficial.

EXPLAINING TECHNIQUES

Clients should fully understand reflexology so they are more comfortable with the procedure. The simplicity of reflexology belies its efficacy, so a knowledge of the subject will give the client confidence in the ability of reflexology to help him or her. But knowledge alone cannot eliminate disease. Reflexology, as a touch technique centered on the feet, is a relatively intimate practice. The receiver must be made to feel comfortable and "safe." He or she will often feel the need to talk and should always feel free to do so. Healing is also an art that requires intuitive skills.

The art of recognizing the roots of a client's problem and working with him or her to overcome this can be learned only through experience, practice, self-knowledge, and constant attentiveness.

It is important to explain to the recipient as much as possible about the treatment and techniques to be used before commencing the actual treatment procedure. This is because there should ideally be no conversation during the massage. Talking gives rise to images forming in the recipient's mind, which in turn cause physical reactions within the body. Muscles tense and heart rate increases.

The art of reflexology requires thorough knowledge of grips,
pressure techniques, relaxation techniques, and a step-by-step
treatment sequence for all the reflexes.

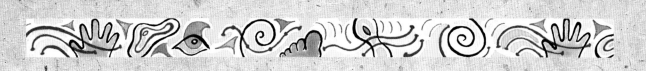

PART THREE

PRACTICAL
RFFLEXOLOGY

11. BASIC TECHNIQUES

The body is reflected on the feet in a three-dimensional form. Organs overlap each other internally and, therefore, the same configuration is found on the feet. Many organs are minute and not reflected on the charts, but all are worked on in the step-by-step treatment sequence.

Many reflexologists propose working one foot completely before moving on to the next. The main objective of the reflexologist is to stimulate all the reflexes on the feet. Since any technique that achieves this result is equally effective, it is up to you to choose which technique works best for you. I have found in my years of practice and teaching that the techniques illustrated on the following pages in this chapter have proved their worth.

The most important aspect of this treatment procedure is that both feet are worked through alternately from toe to heel. This facilitates a natural flow. One foot represents half a body, and since many organs are paired and found on both sides of the body, it would be wrong to complete one foot at a time. This would mean only half an organ is stimulated.

In the remainder of this chapter the basic technique of holding and supporting the foot using the standard support grip is described, followed by the six standard pressure techniques and seven grips used to work the reflexes on the feet. The relaxation sequence generally used at the beginning of a treatment is also described. (References to "right" and "left" feet mean the receiver's right and left, not the practitioner's.)

Once you have mastered the basic techniques, you will be able to apply them in a reflexology treatment described in Chapter 12. A summary chart on pages 146–147 shows the order of treatment and indicates which grips and pressure techniques are used for working each of the different reflexes of the feet.

RIGHT
The feet should be massaged in sequence from toe to heel, alternating feet as you go.

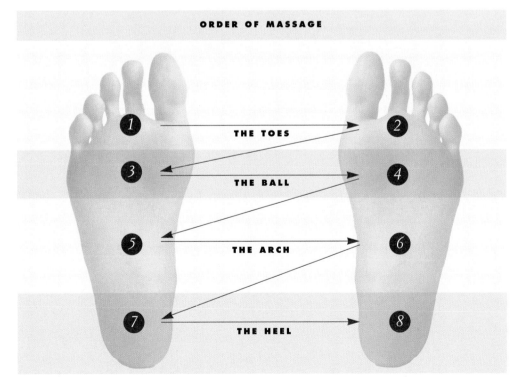

ORDER OF MASSAGE

1 → 2 THE TOES

3 ← 4 THE BALL

5 ← 6 THE ARCH

7 ← 8 THE HEEL

Self-Treatment with Reflexology

Before looking at specific grips and techniques, we will look briefly at the potential for treating yourself using reflexology. Self-treatment can be awkward and arduous, but if you are willing to devote the time and energy to yourself, it is certainly worth the effort.

There are disadvantages to self-treatment. First and foremost, all-important relaxation is impossible to achieve. And second, the vital energy exchange between subject and practitioner – which plays a major role in the success of the treatment – is lacking, since you are both the practitioner and patient at the same time. Self-treatment is, therefore, useful on as a means of preventive treatment, general health care, and first aid (to achieve quick relief from a condition), until you can arrange for professional assistance. This form of self-treatment, although beneficial, could never be as effective as, or replace, professional treatment from a trained practitioner.

Self-treatment can be undertaken by anyone reasonably agile. One should be able to sit comfortably cross-legged or raise one foot onto the opposite knee.

FULL TREATMENT

Sit on a chair or cross-legged on the floor or bed with cushions behind your back. If you are aware which reflexes are out of balance, work specifically on those. Remember, it is difficult to assess your own reflexes accurately. Work slowly and gently through the whole treatment sequence described on pages 148–173.

An alternative is to concentrate treatments on the toes, in which sections of the six main meridians are present. Stimulating these can be extremely beneficial. It is important to be as relaxed as possible, with no tension in the legs.

A full treatment will take approximately an hour, which may be a bit much for many to contemplate. However, treatment of reflex points can be used to relieve headaches, migraines, muscle aches, and other transient conditions. At the end of a treatment always sit or lie back for approximately 15 minutes and relax using the appropriate techniques for breathing.

All six meridians are present in the toe area.

Relaxed feet and ankles are essential.

Learn where specific reflex points are located.

Sit comfortably on the floor if possible, or on a bed.

Wear comfortable, loose clothing.

Sit cross-legged, one foot raised onto opposite knee.

Work on specific reflexes, slowly and gently.

RIGHT
Self-treatment is very beneficial, but you must be reasonably agile to administer it.

Holding the Foot

The first priority for effective reflexology is to learn correct support. Otherwise, the pressure techniques will never be thoroughly mastered. The hands perform complementary functions throughout the treatment. While one hand presses, the other braces and supports or pushes the foot toward the pressure. The hand applying pressure is referred to as the "working hand," the other hand, the "supporting hand." Neither hand should ever be idle.

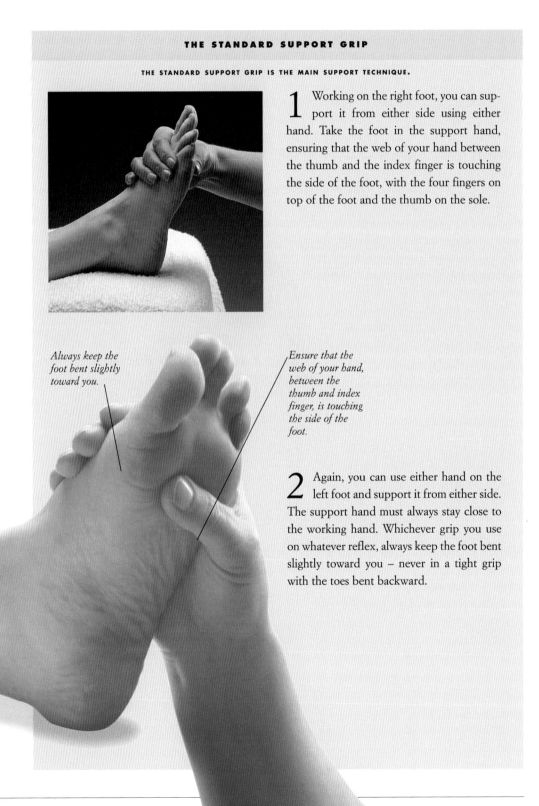

THE STANDARD SUPPORT GRIP

THE STANDARD SUPPORT GRIP IS THE MAIN SUPPORT TECHNIQUE.

1 Working on the right foot, you can support it from either side using either hand. Take the foot in the support hand, ensuring that the web of your hand between the thumb and the index finger is touching the side of the foot, with the four fingers on top of the foot and the thumb on the sole.

Always keep the foot bent slightly toward you.

Ensure that the web of your hand, between the thumb and index finger, is touching the side of the foot.

2 Again, you can use either hand on the left foot and support it from either side. The support hand must always stay close to the working hand. Whichever grip you use on whatever reflex, always keep the foot bent slightly toward you – never in a tight grip with the toes bent backward.

Pressure Techniques

There are six standard pressure techniques for working the reflexes of the feet in conjunction with the grips described on pages 142–145.

ROTATING THUMB TECHNIQUE

THE ROTATING THUMB TECHNIQUE IS THE MOST IMPORTANT TECHNIQUE TO MASTER BECAUSE IT IS USED TO APPLY PRESSURE TO MOST OF THE REFLEXES THROUGHOUT THE TREATMENT PROCEDURE. BEFORE WORKING ON THE FEET, PRACTICE THE ROTATING THUMB TECHNIQUE ON THE PALM OF YOUR HAND UNTIL YOU FEEL COMFORTABLE WITH IT. IT HELPS TO VISUALIZE THE OBJECT BEING WORKED ON (HAND OR FOOT) DIVIDED INTO SMALL SQUARES, WHICH MUST BE SYSTEMATICALLY STIMULATED. ALSO EXERCISE THE THUMBS ON BOTH HANDS TO ENABLE YOU TO WORK EFFICIENTLY, SINCE YOU NEED TO SWITCH HANDS DURING THE TREATMENT SEQUENCE.

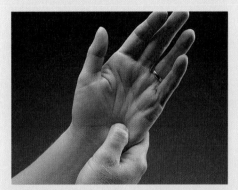

1 Place the four fingers of the working hand on the back of the hand to be worked on, keeping the thumb free to work on the palm. Bend the thumb of the working hand from the first joint to between a 75 and 90 degree angle – the angle must ensure that the thumb nail doesn't dig into the flesh. This is the standard position of the "rotating thumb technique."

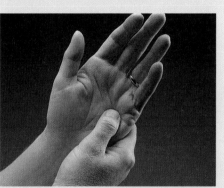

2 Starting at the outside of the hand press with the tip of the thumb and rotate it, clockwise or anticlockwise. Keep the pressure firm and constant and *stay on the visualized square.* Two or three rotations are sufficient. The basic movement is: press in, rotate, lift, move. The amount of pressure or number of rotations depends on the practitioner and client.

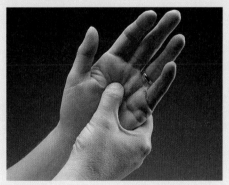

3 Lift the thumb, move to the next point and repeat the procedure. Apply pressure and rotation to each square. Movement must be small, leaving no space between each point. More pressure can be applied with a bent thumb than a flat thumb. Allow 1in. between the thumb and first finger for easy rotations.

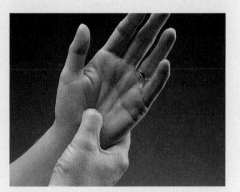

4 The most visible rotation must be at the second thumb joint – where the metacarpals of the hand join the phalanges of the thumb. Two basic tenets for ease in executing this technique are to keep the thumb bent and the shoulders down. There should be little strain on the arm muscles, elbows, neck, and shoulders.

FINGER TECHNIQUE 1

THIS TECHNIQUE IS USED ON THE SIDES AND TOPS OF THE TOES.

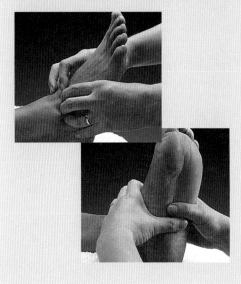

1 Place the index finger on one side and the thumb on the other side of the toe to be worked on. "Rub" the toe, moving the fingers gently back and forth in opposite directions. Move from toe to toe using this technique on each.

FINGER TECHNIQUE 2

THIS IS USED ON THE FALLOPIAN TUBES/VAS DEFERENS AND LYMPHATIC REFLEXES.

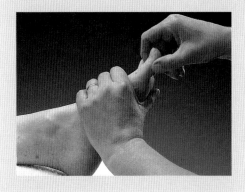

1 Place your hands on either side of the foot, with the four fingers just underneath the ankle bone and the thumbs on the sole. The index and middle fingers are the working tools; the middle finger is usually placed on top of the index finger to create extra leverage.

2 With the fingers, press in, rotate, lift and move as with the rotating thumb. Move the fingers gradually, point by point up both sides of the foot until your fingers meet at the center on top of the foot. Each movement should be slight.

FINGER TECHNIQUE 3

USE THESE RELAXING TECHNIQUES AS PART OF THE WINDING DOWN STAGE OF THE TREATMENT.

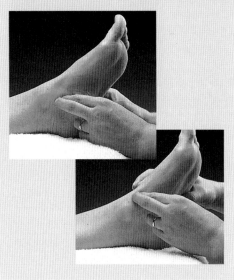

1 Place your hands on either side of the foot, thumbs on the sole forming the support and the four fingers of each hand on top. Starting from the ankle joint, exert deep, smooth pressure massaging down the foot toward the toes. You can improvise on this technique as long as you ensure that you massage well.

2 Then, work the sides of the feet using a criss-cross movement with your thumbs. Cream or oil can be used at this stage to facilitate easy movement.

PINCH TECHNIQUE

THE PINCH TECHNIQUE IS USED TO STIMULATE THE KIDNEY AND BLADDER MERIDIANS. WITH THIS TECHNIQUE IT DOES NOT MATTER WHICH HAND YOU USE TO SUPPORT OR WHICH YOU USE TO WORK WITH. HOWEVER, IT IS IMPORTANT TO HOLD THE FOOT FIRMLY SO THAT THE PATIENT FEELS SECURE AND, THEREFORE, ABLE TO RELAX.

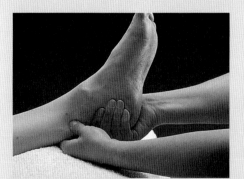

1 The support hand cups the foot holding the area below the outer ankle bone with the thumb and below the inner ankle bone with the four fingers. Locate the Achilles tendon at the back of the heel with both the thumb and the index finger of the working hand.

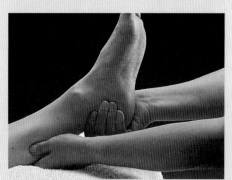

2 With the thumb and index finger of the working hand, move up and down the tendon pinching it gently.

KNEAD TECHNIQUE

THIS IS A RELATIVELY EASY TECHNIQUE, MUCH LIKE KNEADING BREAD. IT IS USED FOR WORKING THE REFLEXES IN THE HEEL – THE PELVIC AND SCIATIC NERVE REFLEXES. THE HEEL AREA IS USUALLY RATHER TOUGH AND, THEREFORE, NEEDS MORE PRESSURE FOR EFFECTIVE STIMULATION.

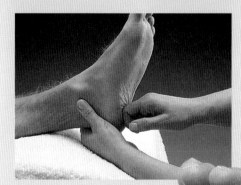

1 Cup the back of the ankle in the palm of the support hand, with the thumb around one side of the ankle and the four fingers around the other side. Keep the heel area free. Make a fist with the working hand.

Ensure that the foot is well supported by cupping the back of the ankle.

2 Using the second joint of the fingers of the working hand "knead" the heels as you would dough.

THESE ARE THE MAIN BASIC FINGER AND THUMB TECHNIQUES USED IN THE TREATMENT PROCEDURE. SINCE ONE OF THE MAIN BENEFITS OF REFLEXOLOGY IS THE RELAXATION ASPECT, IT IS ALSO IMPORTANT TO BECOME FAMILIAR WITH A FEW BASIC RELAXATION TECHNIQUES.

"Knead" the heel as you would dough.

Relaxation Techniques

ACHILLES TENDON STRETCH

USE THIS TECHNIQUE TO STRETCH THE BACK OF THE LEG, RELEASING TENSION, AND THEREBY INCREASING
MOBILITY IN THE ANKLE. THE STRETCHING ALSO STIMULATES CIRCULATION AND FOOT FLEXION.

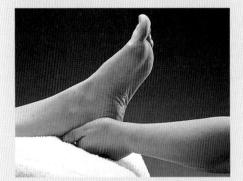

1 If working on the left foot, use your right hand as the support, and vice versa for the right foot. Cup the heel of the foot firmly but gently, so it rests in your support hand, and you take the full weight of the foot. Curve your fingers around the outside of the heel and your thumb around the inside.

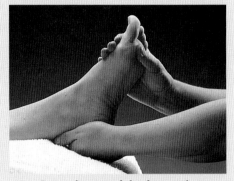

2 Grasp the top of the foot in the standard support grip (see page 132), near the base of the toes, thumb underneath, fingers on top. Be careful not to grip too tightly. Your hand should be relaxed.

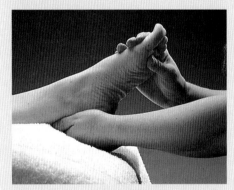

3 Pull the top of the foot toward you. Do not force the heel back, but allow it to move slightly backward naturally.

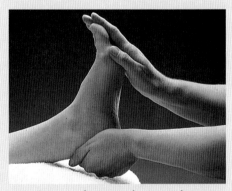

4 Reverse the procedure, gently easing the heel toward you so that the sole of the foot stretches out, stretching the Achilles tendon. As you do this flex the foot. Repeat this technique three times on each foot.

Feet raised and ready for treatment

Ankles loose and relaxed

ANKLE ROTATION

THIS TECHNIQUE AFFECTS THE ENTIRE AREA OF THE HIP JOINT AND TAILBONE, RELAXES THE ANUS AND SURROUNDING AREA AND AFFECTS ALL THE LOWER BACK MUSCLES. BECAUSE A RELAXED ANKLE INDICATES A RELAXED BODY, IT IS ESSENTIAL THAT THE CLIENT FEELS SECURE. DO NOT FORCE THE FOOT INTO EXAGGERATED CIRCLES; MANEUVER IT SLOWLY AND GENTLY ONLY AS FAR AS IS COMFORTABLE FOR THE RECEIVER. YOU MUST CARRY OUT THIS MOVEMENT SMOOTHLY.

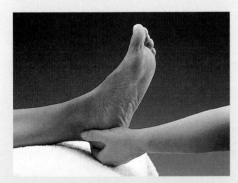

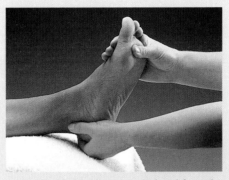

1 Cup the back of the ankle of the left foot in the palm of your left (support) hand, with the thumb on the inside of the ankle and the fingers on the outside. Ensure a firm but not tight grasp so that the client feels secure and relaxed.

2 Working with your right hand from the outside of the foot, grasp the foot at the base of the toes in the standard support grip *(see page 132)*. Hold the foot using equal pressure with both hands.

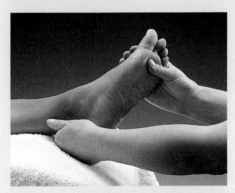

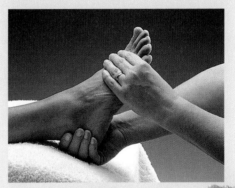

3 Use the hand holding the ankle joint as a pivot, and rotate the foot with the right hand in a 360-degree circle, first clockwise a few times, then anticlockwise.

4 Work the right foot the same way, using the palm of your right hand to support the ankle and using your left hand to work the foot.

BELOW
During a reflexology treatment, the client should be seated in a relaxed position with the feet raised.

LOOSEN ANKLES

USE THIS TECHNIQUE TO LOOSEN AND RELAX BOTH ANKLE JOINTS. THE FLEXIBILITY OF THE ANKLE JOINTS REFLECTS THE
FLEXIBILITY OF ALL THE JOINTS IN THE WHOLE BODY – RELAXED ANKLES INDICATE A RELAXED BODY.

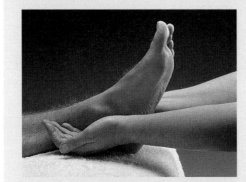 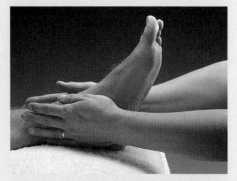

1 Position your hands either side of the ankle bone so that the base of each palm lies above the sides of the heel, behind the ankle bone. The outer edges of your hands should rest behind the ankle joint. Cup your hands so that your palms cover the ankle joint, which serves as the pivot point.

2 Move your hands rapidly backward and forward in opposite directions to each other, keeping them cupped over the ankle bones. The foot will shake from side to side when this movement is correctly executed. Continue using this technique until the ankle feels fully relaxed.

SIDE TO SIDE

THE SIDE TO SIDE TECHNIQUE IS OFTEN USED AS PART OF A RELAXATION TREATMENT. IT BENEFITS THE CIRCULATION BY
VIGOROUSLY SHAKING THE FOOT, AND EASES TENDERNESS. MOST IMPORTANT, IT RELAXES THE ANKLE AND CALF MUSCLES. ONCE
THESE ARE TOTALLY RELAXED, THE WHOLE BODY WILL ALSO BE RELAXED.

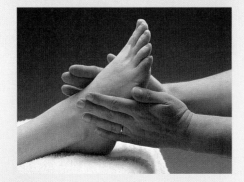

1 Place your palms on either side of the foot just above the ankles. Keep your hands as relaxed and loose as possible. Do not force the foot to rotate farther than is comfortable for the client. Roll the foot from side to side by gently moving it back and forth between your hands, which move up and down in opposite directions from each other.

Roll the foot back and forth between your hands.

Move your hands gradually up the sides of the foot.

2 Move your hands gradually up the side of the foot until the entire foot is worked. This is usually executed slowly to release tension, relax the edges of the ankle and calf, and stimulate the whole foot.

SPINAL TWIST

THE SPINAL TWIST IS THE MOST RELAXING TECHNIQUE AND SHOULD BE EXECUTED ON BOTH FEET. THIS EFFECTIVE TENSION
REDUCER IS ENJOYED BY MOST CLIENTS. IF YOU ARE WORKING ON THE RIGHT FOOT, THE RIGHT HAND IS THE SUPPORT AND THE
LEFT HAND IS THE WORKING HAND, AND VICE VERSA ON THE LEFT FOOT.

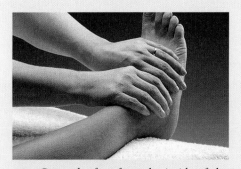

1 Grasp the foot from the inside of the instep using both hands, fingers on top, thumbs on the sole – the web between the thumb and the index finger on the spinal reflex, with index fingers touching.

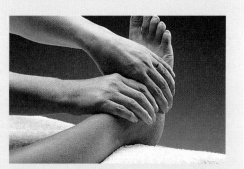

2 The hand close to the ankle will provide the support. The hand nearest the toes will execute the twisting action. The hands should be used as a unit, keeping the fingers together and the hands touching.

The twisting action is carried out by the hand nearest the toes.

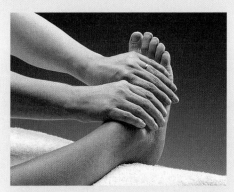

3 Keeping the support hand steady, twist the working hand up and down. The support hand must remain completely stationary at all times.

4 Move back toward the toes and repeat the twisting action.

The hand close to the ankle provides support.

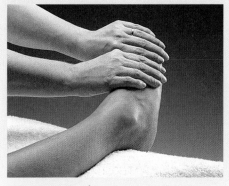

5 Continue this movement (grip, twist, reposition, grip, twist, reposition) working in small stages along the entire length of the foot.

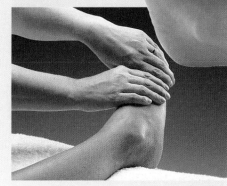

6 Your final position is the neck reflex area at the base of the big toe. Do not twist both hands at the same time. Keep the support hand still while the working hand twists. Repeat this technique on the left foot.

WRINGING THE FOOT

THIS TECHNIQUE IS USED PURELY TO RELAX THE CLIENT'S BODY FROM THE NECK DOWN TO THE BASE OF THE SPINE. IT DOES NOT CONCENTRATE ON ANY REFLEX POINTS; THEREFORE, IT IS AN EXCELLENT COMPLEMENT TO OTHER RELAXATION TECHNIQUES. THIS TECHNIQUE IS SIMILAR TO THE SPINAL TWIST EXCEPT BOTH HANDS MOVE IN THE WRINGING MOTION.

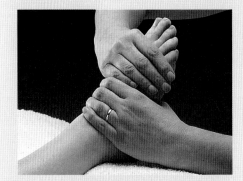

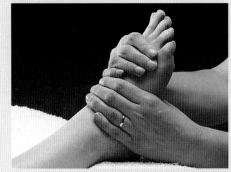

1 Grasp the foot in both hands as you would a wet towel and wring gently. Each hand must twist in opposite directions.

2 Your elbows should fly up and move when you do this. Move your hands gradually up to "wring" its entire length.

ROTATE ALL TOES

THE PRINCIPLE HERE IS THE SAME AS THE ANKLE ROTATION. IT IS A RELAXATION TECHNIQUE THAT NOT ONLY INCREASES FLEXIBILITY OF THE TOES, BUT RELEASES TENSION AND LOOSENS MUSCLES IN THE NECK AND SHOULDER LINE. HOWEVER, DO NOT USE THIS TECHNIQUE ON CLIENTS WHO SUFFER FROM OSTEOPOROSIS OR BRITTLE BONE DISEASE.

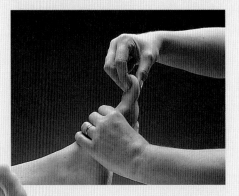

1 Begin with the big toe. Firmly hold the base of the toe you are going to rotate with the thumb and fingers of your support hand (left hand for left foot, right hand for right foot) in the standard support grip (see page 132). With your working hand hold the toe close to the base joint (metatarsal/phalange joint), with your thumb below and your index and third finger on top.

Gently "lift" the toe.

Stabilize the toe at the base with the support hand.

2 Now gently "lift" the toe in its joint with a slightly upward pull and rotate in 360-degree circles, clockwise then anticlockwise a few times. Movements must be gentle but firm, the support hand stabilizing the toe at the base as it is worked on. Repeat this procedure on each toe of one foot in turn, then perform the technique on the other foot.

SOLAR PLEXUS

USE THIS TECHNIQUE FOR CLIENTS WHO EXHIBIT SYMPTOMS OF STRESS. THE SOLAR PLEXUS IS REFERRED TO AS THE "NERVE SWITCHBOARD" OF THE BODY, SINCE IT IS THE MAIN STORAGE AREA FOR STRESS. APPLYING PRESSURE TO THIS REFLEX WILL ALWAYS BRING ABOUT A FEELING OF RELAXATION. THIS TECHNIQUE IS OFTEN USED AS PART OF A SERIES OF RELAXATION METHODS AT THE BEGINNING OF A TREATMENT, BUT CAN BE USED AT ANY TIME DURING TREATMENT IF NECESSARY. PRESSURE APPLIED TO THE SOLAR PLEXUS REFLEX IS ALSO USED TO RELAX A CLIENT AT THE END OF A TREATMENT SEQUENCE.

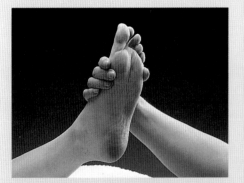

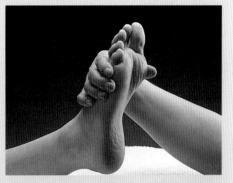

1 To locate the solar plexus reflex, grasp the top of the foot at the metatarsal area at the sides of the foot level with the ball. Squeeze the sides of the foot gently.

2 A depression will appear on the sole of the foot at the center of the diaphragm line – the midpoint of the base of the ball of the foot. This is the solar plexus reflex.

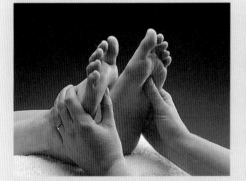

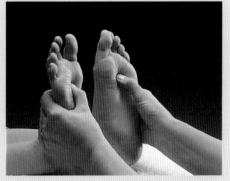

3 Apply this technique to both feet simultaneously. Take the left foot in your right hand and the right foot in your left hand, fingers on top, thumbs on the sole – from the outside of each foot. Place the tips of your thumbs on the solar plexus reflex.

4 Ask the client to inhale slowly as you press in on this point and exhale as you release pressure. Do not lose contact with the foot.

Press the reflex in time with the client's breathing. Never lose contact with the foot.

Place your fingers on top and your thumb on the sole of the foot.

5 Continue to press and release pressure on the reflex while the client inhales and exhales a few times until the client is totally relaxed.

Grips

The reflexologist must acquire a good supporting technique for the treatment to be completely successful. It is important to support the client's foot firmly so that it does not roll around, thus enabling you to execute movements with your working hand on the correct part of the foot. Moreover, the client must feel secure and able to relax totally. A good supporting technique using the grips described below means that the reflexologist is in control.

REFLEXES
WORKED WITH
GRIP

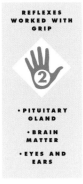

1

• SINUSES

• CHRONIC
EYES AND
EARS

• BRONCHI,
LUNGS, AND
HEART

GRIP 1

GRIP 1 IS USED TO WORK THE REFLEXES OF THE TOES AND BALL OF THE FOOT.

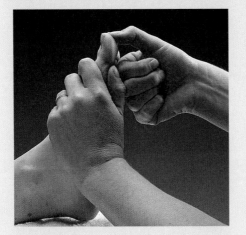

Make a clenched fist with your working hand, keeping the thumb free. The fist of the working hand will provide additional support on the sole of the foot. The rotating thumb technique (see page 133) is used to exert pressure on the reflex points. Your support hand is in the standard support position (see page 132) close to the working hand. With grip 1, the left hand is usually the support hand and the right hand the worker.

REFLEXES
WORKED WITH
GRIP

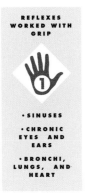

2

• PITUITARY
GLAND

• BRAIN
MATTER

• EYES AND
EARS

GRIP 2

THE TOES ARE ALSO WORKED USING GRIP 2.

For this technique you can use either hand to support and work the foot. Your support hand holds the foot in the standard support grip (see page 132) close to the base of the toes. With your working hand, clasp the foot from above. Place the fingers on the top of the foot at the toes, pointing toward the ankle. The thumb is then positioned at the back of the toes in order to work under them.

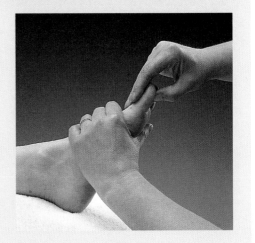

GRIP 3

SOMETIMES IT IS DIFFICULT TO LOCATE AND STIMULATE THE PITUITARY GLAND USING THE TECHNIQUE SHOWN IN GRIP 2, BECAUSE IT IS EASY TO MISS THE REFLEX USING ONLY THE TIP OF YOUR THUMB. GRIP 2 IS AN ALTERNATIVE TO GRIP 2 IN SUCH CASES.

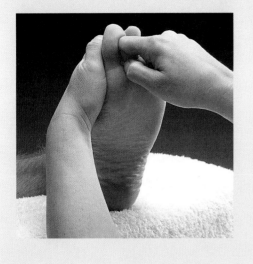

Bend the index finger of your working hand at the second joint and use this as you would your thumb in grip 2. Find the reflex, press in, rotate clockwise and anti-clockwise a few times, then release the pressure when you feel the reflex has been sufficiently stimulated. You will know when this point has been reached because the client will no longer feel discomfort when the reflex is pressed. This comes with experience of practicing the technique.

REFLEXES
WORKED WITH
GRIP

3

• PITUITARY
GLAND

GRIP 4

THIS GRIP IS BENEFICIAL FOR WORKING THE REFLEXES OF THE UPPER LYMPHATIC SYSTEM. HERE, YOUR LEFT HAND IS THE SUPPORT HAND AND YOUR RIGHT HAND THE WORKING HAND ON BOTH FEET.

1 Cup the sole of the foot at the arch in the palm of your support hand. The thumb of your working hand provides support on the sole of the foot, and the index finger is responsible for the rotations on the top of the foot. Place the middle finger of your working hand on top of the index finger for greater pressure. Reach between the toes until the web between the thumb and index finger touches the web between the big and second toe. Using the rotation movement *(see page 133)*, work point by point back toward the webs.

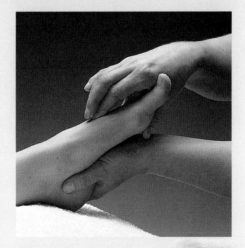

REFLEXES
WORKED WITH
GRIP

4

• UPPER
LYMPHATICS

Apply a pinching pressure to the webs between the toes.

2 When you get to the webs, apply a tight, pinching pressure on them. The webs are important lymphatic reflexes. Repeat this pinching pressure between each toe, using the grooves between the metatarsal bones as guidelines. Repeat the complete technique on the other foot.

Cup the arch of the foot securely.

REFLEXES
WORKED WITH
GRIP

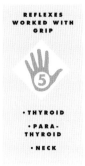

5

• THYROID
• PARA-
THYROID
• NECK

GRIP 5

GRIP 5 IS USED FOR WORKING THE THYROID REFLEX. THIS REFLEX COVERS THE ENTIRE AREA OF THE BALL OF THE FOOT AT THE BASE OF THE BIG TOE. TO ACHIEVE SUFFICIENT STIMULATION, YOU MUST GET RIGHT INTO THE BONE AT THE BASE OF THE BALL AND PRESS "UP AND UNDER." IN GRIP 5, YOUR ELBOWS MUST MOVE OUT AND UP INTO THE AIR TO FACILITATE THE ANGLE NECESSARY TO GET RIGHT INTO THE THYROID REFLEX. IF WORKING ON THE LEFT FOOT, THE SUPPORT HAND WILL BE YOUR LEFT HAND AND THE WORKING HAND WILL BE YOUR RIGHT, AND VICE VERSA.

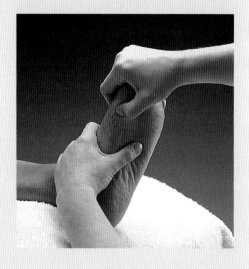

With your support hand, hold the foot in the standard support grip *(see page 132)* just below the ball of the foot. The fingers of your working hand grasp the foot from the inside of the instep, fingers on top of the foot from approximately halfway down the big toe, and the thumb poised to work the important half-moon section of the thyroid reflex at the base of the ball. With the thumb, press in and up to get right to the bone and use the rotating thumb technique *(see page 133)* to work around the half-circle of the ball, up to the neck reflex, and then cover the section at the base of the big toe.

REFLEXES
WORKED WITH
GRIP

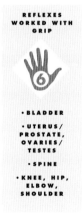

6

• BLADDER
• UTERUS/
PROSTATE,
OVARIES/
TESTES
• SPINE
• KNEE, HIP,
ELBOW,
SHOULDER

GRIP 6

THIS GRIP IS USED MAINLY FOR WORKING ON THE SIDES OF THE FEET – THE SPINE AND BLADDER REFLEXES ON THE INNER FOOT, AND THE KNEE, HIP, ELBOW, AND SHOULDER REFLEXES ON THE OUTER FOOT. WORK THE FEET ALTERNATELY.

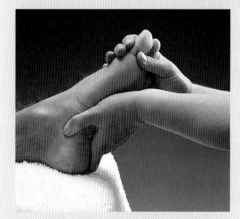

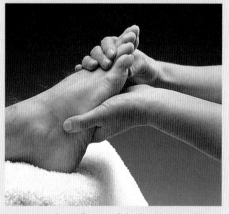

1 For this grip, the foot is cupped in the palm of your working hand, the sole of the foot resting in the palm, leaving the thumb free to execute the rotating thumb technique *(see page 133)*. The support hand is in the standard support grip *(see page 132)* at the base of the toes. To work the reflexes of the spine and bladder on the inner foot, support the left foot with your right hand and work with your left thumb. Change hands to work these reflexes on the inner right foot.

2 For the reflexes of the knee, hip, elbow, and shoulder on the outer foot, support the right foot with your right hand and work with the left. Change hands to work on the left foot.

GRIP 7

REFLEXES
WORKED WITH
GRIP

7

• LIVER/GALL
BLADDER

• STOMACH,
PANCREAS,
DUODENUM,
SPLEEN

• SMALL
INTESTINE,
ILEO-CECAL
VALVE,
APPENDIX

• LARGE
INTESTINE

• KIDNEY,
ADRENALS,
URETERS

THIS TECHNIQUE MAY SOUND SLIGHTLY CONFUSING AT FIRST, BUT IT DEFINITELY FACILITATES A SMOOTH AND FLOWING TECHNIQUE FOR WORKING THE DIGESTIVE AREA. TO PERFORM GRIP 7 IMAGINE EACH FOOT IS DIVIDED IN HALF VERTICALLY. THE OBJECT IS TO WORK HORIZONTALLY ACROSS BOTH FEET AS IF THEY ARE A SINGLE UNIT TOWARD THE IMAGINARY VERTICAL LINE, USING IT AS THE POINT AT WHICH YOU SWAP WORKING HANDS. POSITION YOURSELF SO THAT YOU ARE ABLE TO SWIVEL IN YOUR SEAT; YOU SHOULD NOT WORK THE FOOT "STRAIGHT ON."

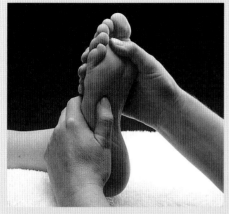

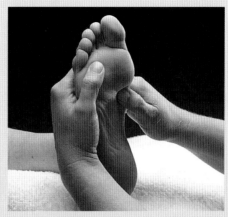

1 Support the right foot with your right hand in the standard support grip *(see page 132)* at the base of the toes. Work the outer side of the sole of the foot with your left thumb. The pressure is, as usual, exerted with the rotating thumb *(see page 133)*. The liver and gall bladder reflexes above the waistline are worked here.

2 Support the right foot with your left hand and work the inner side of the sole of the foot with your right thumb. The stomach, pancreas, duodenum, kidney, and adrenal reflexes above the waistline are worked here.

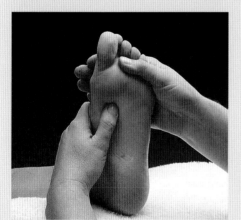

Use the standard support grip at the base of the foot.

Work horizontally across both feet.

3 Move on to the left foot. Support the left foot with your right hand and work the inner side of the sole of the foot with your left thumb. Again, the stomach, pancreas, duodenum, kidney, and adrenal reflexes above the waistline are worked here.

4 Support the left foot with your left hand and work the outer side of the sole of the foot with your right thumb. The spleen reflex is worked here.

The treatment sequence is divided into the same main areas as mentioned in "Mapping the Feet."

Do not forget – the feet are worked alternatively from toe to heel, organ by organ.

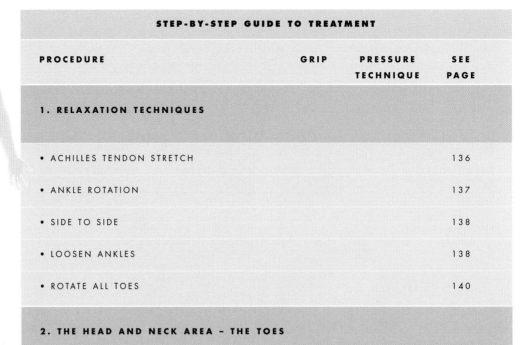

STEP-BY-STEP GUIDE TO TREATMENT			
PROCEDURE	**GRIP**	**PRESSURE TECHNIQUE**	**SEE PAGE**
1. RELAXATION TECHNIQUES			
• ACHILLES TENDON STRETCH			136
• ANKLE ROTATION			137
• SIDE TO SIDE			138
• LOOSEN ANKLES			138
• ROTATE ALL TOES			140
2. THE HEAD AND NECK AREA – THE TOES			
• SINUSES	①	⬙	150
• PITUITARY GLAND	② OR ③	⬙	151
• BRAIN MATTER	②	⬙	151
• EYES AND EARS	②	⬙	152
• SIDES AND TOPS OF TOES		⬙	153
• CHRONIC EYES AND EARS	①	⬙	154
• UPPER LYMPHATICS	④		155
3. THE THORACIC AREA – THE BALL OF THE FOOT			
• BRONCHI, LUNGS, AND HEART	①	⬙	157
• THYROID, PARATHYROID, AND NECK	⑤	⬙	158
• DIAPHRAGM	①	⬙	159
4. THE ABDOMINAL AREA – THE ARCH OF THE FOOT			
• LIVER AND GALL BLADDER	⑦	⬙	161
• STOMACH, PANCREAS, DUODENUM, & SPLEEN	⑦	⬙	162
• SMALL INTESTINE/ILEO-CECAL VALVE	⑦	⬙	163
• APPENDIX	⑦	⬙	163

146

STEP-BY-STEP GUIDE TO TREATMENT

PROCEDURE	GRIP	PRESSURE TECHNIQUE	SEE PAGE
4. THE ABDOMINAL AREA – THE ARCH (CONTINUED)			
• LARGE INTESTINE	7		164
• KIDNEYS AND ADRENALS	7		165
• URETERS AND BLADDER	6 AND 2		166
5. THE PELVIC AREA – THE HEEL OF THE FOOT			
• PELVIS AND SCIATIC NERVE		OR	167
6. THE REPRODUCTIVE AREA – THE ANKLE			
• UTERUS, OVARIES, PROSTATE, AND TESTES	6		168
• FALLOPIAN TUBES, AND VAS DEFERENS	6	OR	169
7. THE SPINE – THE INNER FOOT			
• SPINAL TWIST		RELAXATION	139
• SPINE	6		170
8. THE OUTER BODY – THE OUTER FOOT			
• KNEE, HIP, ELBOW, AND SHOULDER	6		171
9. CIRCULATION AND BREASTS – THE TOP OF THE FOOT			
• BREASTS AND CIRCULATION			172
10. RELAXATION TECHNIQUES			
• KIDNEY AND BLADDER MERIDIANS			172
• SOLAR PLEXUS DEEP BREATHING			173

12. THE TREATMENT SEQUENCE IN DETAIL

This description of the treatment sequence is included to give you a more comprehensive grasp of how to proceed through the full treatment easily and fluidly.

Relaxation

The first step in the treatment procedure is to relax the client, release tension from the ankles, and loosen the feet. Begin with the relaxation techniques in the order shown below. Following this the receiver should feel primed for the full treatment. Whichever grip you use on whatever reflex, always hold the foot in a firm but gentle grip, and keep the foot bent slightly toward you.

ACHILLES TENDON STRETCH

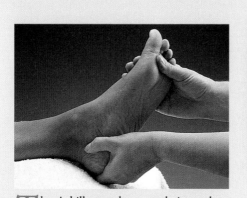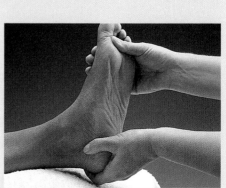

The Achilles tendon stretch is used to release tension and stretch the back of the leg. For a full description of the technique, *see page 136.*

ANKLE ROTATION

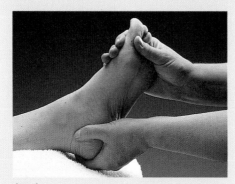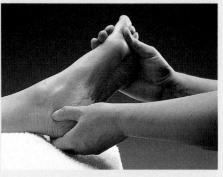

The ankle is rotated clockwise then anti-clockwise, to relax the area surrounding the anus and lower back muscles. For a full description of the technique, *see page 137.*

SIDE TO SIDE

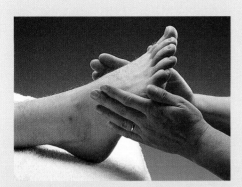 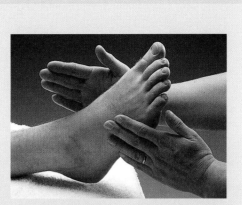

The side to side technique involves rolling the foot from side to side, which stimulates the circulation and relaxes the ankle and calf muscles. For a full description of the technique, *see page 138*.

LOOSEN ANKLES

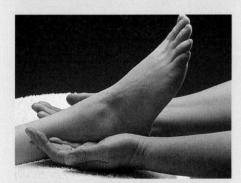 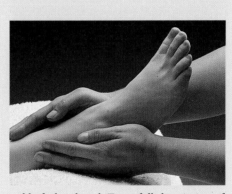

Relaxing the ankle will help relax all the joints in the body. The foot is shaken from side to side in this technique until the ankle feels relaxed. For a full description of the technique, *see page 138*.

ROTATE ALL TOES

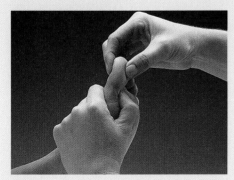 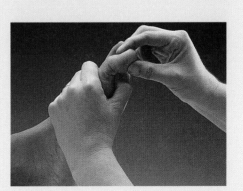

The rotate all toes technique works in a similar way to the ankle rotation and releases tension and loosens muscles in the neck and shoulder. For a full description of the technique, *see page 140*.

The Head and Neck Area – the Toes

The toes represent the head and neck area. Reflexes found here include the pituitary gland, pineal gland, hypothalamus, brain matter, eyes and ears, sinuses. Babies respond well to stimulation of these reflexes, which should be light in pressure and short in duration. Children and the elderly also benefit from this treatment, but again, use light pressure. Every person's sensitivities are different: make sure that you never exceed an individual's pain threshold.

SINUSES

THE SINUS REFLEXES ARE SITUATED ON THE TOPS OF THE TOES. WORK THESE FROM THE BIG TO SMALL TOE, FIRST ONE FOOT, THEN THE OTHER. THESE PICTURES SHOW A REFLEXOLOGIST WORKING ON A BABY'S FOOT WHEN THE GRIPS AND TECHNIQUES WILL HAVE TO BE ADAPTED TO THE NEEDS OF THE CHILD. HOLD THE FOOT LOOSELY SO THAT IT CAN BE PULLED AWAY AND MAKE YOUR PRESSURE LIGHT AND YOUR TREATMENT SHORT. REMEMBER THAT YOUR THUMB WILL COVER A LARGE AREA OF THE TOES WITH JUST ONE ROTATION TECHNIQUE.

TOES

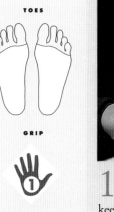

GRIP

PRESSURE TECHNIQUE

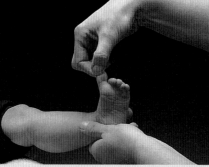

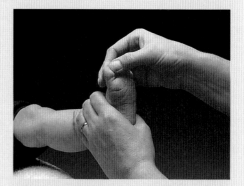

1 Using grip 1 *(see page 142)* make a clenched fist with your working hand, keeping the thumb free. Your left hand will be the support hand and your right hand will be the working hand.

2 Start working on the big toe, applying the thumb rotation technique *(see page 133)* – press in with the thumb, rotate it, and lift and move it to the next position.

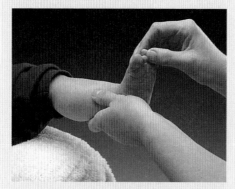

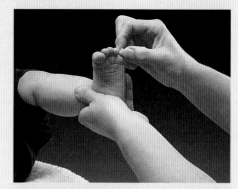

3 The area to cover on each toe would be the equivalent of three to five small "squares" (mentioned in the practice exercises on *page 133*), depending on the size of the toe being worked on.

4 Hold each toe individually with the support hand as you work them to prevent the toes from moving and bending. The fist of the working hand will provide additional support on the sole of the foot.

PITUITARY GLAND, BRAIN MATTER, EYES AND EARS

THE PITUITARY GLAND REFLEX IS SITUATED WITHIN THE BRAIN REFLEX ON THE BIG TOE. THE EXACT POINT MUST BE LOCATED AND INDIVIDUALLY WORKED ON TO STIMULATE THE ENDOCRINE SYSTEM. TO PINPOINT THIS REFLEX, LOOK CLOSELY AT THE PRINT OF THE BIG TOE. THE REFLEX POINT IS SITUATED WHERE THE "WHORL" OF THE PRINT CONVERGES INTO THE CENTRAL POINT. IT OFTEN REQUIRES A LITTLE SEARCHING, BUT IS USUALLY FOUND TOWARD THE INNER SIDE OF THE TOE. SOMETIMES THIS REFLEX IS CLEAR AS A SMALL MOUND. A SHARP PAIN MARKS THE SITE OF THIS REFLEX, SO THERE WILL BE NO MISTAKING IT.

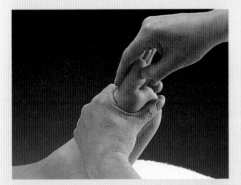

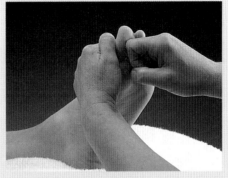

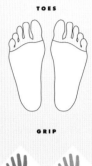

1 Locate the pituitary reflex with the tip of the thumb of your working hand (shown above). Press in with the thumb, rotate and lift. Work this reflex on both feet. Make sure the supporting hand is supporting the toes to prevent them from moving.

2 Alternatively, if you have trouble locating and working the pituitary gland reflex with grip 2, use grip 3 (shown above). You can use either hand to support and work the foot.

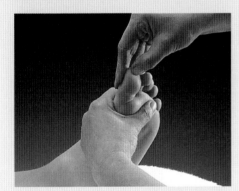

3 Return to the big toe of the foot worked on first, and work the brain reflex area (shown above). Cover the entire area to the base of the big toe using this technique.

After working the brain reflex move on to the eye and ear reflex.

Use either hand to support the foot.

4 Then proceed to work on the eye and ear reflexes on the four toes of the same foot *(see page 152)*, before moving to the other foot to repeat this procedure.

151

EYES AND EARS

THE EYE REFLEXES ARE SITUATED ON THE CUSHIONS OF THE SECOND AND THIRD TOES; THE EAR REFLEXES ON THE CUSHIONS OF THE FOURTH AND FIFTH TOES. IMAGINE THE CUSHIONS OF THE TOES AS INVERTED TRIANGLES. THE THUMB MUST WORK ON THE THREE POINTS OF THE TRIANGLE ON THE CUSHIONS – TWO ABOVE AND ONE BELOW.

TOES

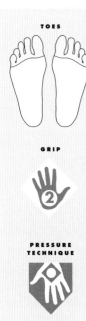

GRIP

PRESSURE TECHNIQUE

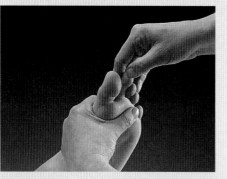

1 Using the standard support grip *(see page 132)* and grip 2 *(see page 142)*. Work the eye reflexes on the second and third toes.

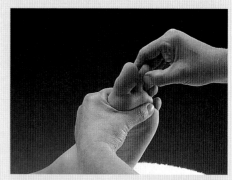

2 Work the "above" points of the triangle using the thumb of your working hand. Then work the "below" point.

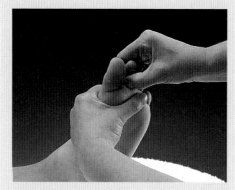

4 Move on to the ear reflexes on the cushions of the fourth and fifth toes and work in the same way. Always support the toes well while you are working on them to prevent them from bending.

3 Then without breaking the flow, continue with the rotating thumb technique down the back of the toe to the base joint (metatarsal/phalange joint).

Always support the toes well to prevent them from bending.

The ear reflexes are found on the fourth and fifth toes.

SIDES AND TOPS OF TOES

THIS TECHNIQUE IS AN EXCELLENT WAY OF STIMULATING THE FLOW OF CH'I (ENERGY) TO THE TOES AND TO THE HEAD
AND NECK REFLEXES. MOST IMPORTANT, THE SIX MAIN MERIDIANS WILL BE STIMULATED.

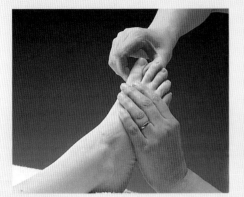

1 Your support hand is in the standard support grip *(see page 132)* at the base of the toes. With your working hand execute finger technique 1 *(see page 134)*. Place the index finger on one side and the thumb on the other side of the toe to be worked on.

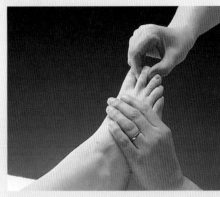

2 Imagine each toe as square in shape. Ensure that both sides and the top of each toe are worked thoroughly.

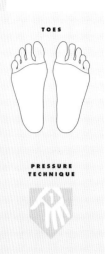

TOES

PRESSURE
TECHNIQUE

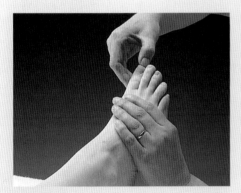

3 "Rub" the toe, moving the fingers gently backwards and forwards in opposite directions.

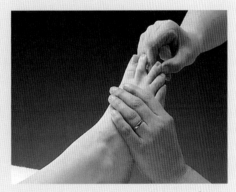

4 It is important to massage each toe thoroughly to ensure that the blood supply is stimulated.

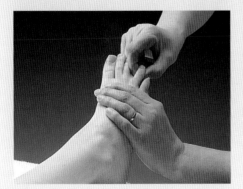

5 This technique also stimulates the head and neck reflexes.

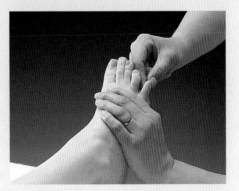

6 When all the toes have been treated, the six main meridians will all have been stimulated.

CHRONIC EYES AND EARS

THESE REFLEXES ARE SITUATED ON THE SOLE OF THE FOOT ALONG THE BASE OF THE FOUR TOES. THE EYE REFLEXES ARE FOUND ON THE SECOND AND THIRD TOES; THE EAR REFLEXES ARE ON THE FOURTH AND FIFTH TOES. THIS AREA ALSO INCLUDES REFLEXES TO THE EUSTACHIAN TUBE, WHICH RUNS FROM THE BACK OF THE NOSE TO THE EAR. THE EUSTACHIAN TUBE REGULATES THE AIR PRESSURE IN THE EAR – THIS IS WHAT HAPPENS WHEN YOUR EAR "POPS."

TOES

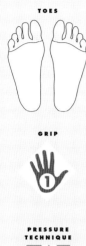

GRIP

PRESSURE TECHNIQUE

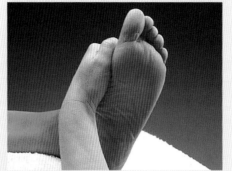

1 If you bend the toes fractionally forward a distinct "shelf" will be visible at the base of the toes. This is the section you will work on. On the left foot, your left hand supports from the inside of the foot and the right hand works from the outside; on the right foot, the left hand supports from the outside of the foot while the right hand works from the inside.

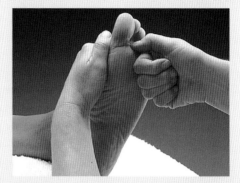

2 To work on these reflexes use the standard support grip (see page 132) and grip 1 (see page 142). Make a fist with your working hand, which will support the sole of the foot, keeping the thumb free. Support the foot with the four fingers and thumb of your supporting hand on the top of the foot.

The four fingers and thumb support the top of the foot.

Work along the shelf at the base of the toes.

Use the rotating thumb technique to work the reflexes.

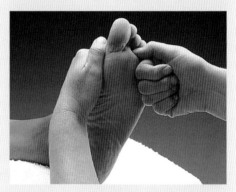

3 Use the rotating thumb technique (see page 133) to work the reflexes along the shelf. Move from point to point along the shelf starting at the second toe.

4 Move all the way along the shelf to the fifth toe and then back again. Repeat this procedure on the other foot.

UPPER LYMPHATICS

ALTHOUGH THE MOST IMPORTANT LYMPHATIC REFLEXES ARE LOCATED IN THE WEBS BETWEEN THE TOES, THE ENTIRE AREA ON THE TOP OF THE FOOT – FROM THE ANKLE JOINT TO THE WEBS – MUST BE WORKED ON FOR OPTIMUM STIMULATION.

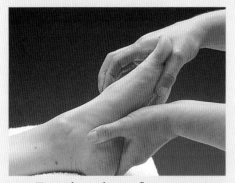

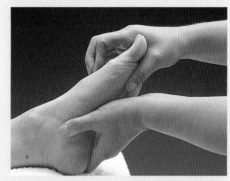

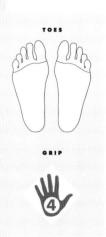

TOES

GRIP

1 To work on these reflexes, use grip 4 working from the ankle joint to webs *(see page 143)*. You can use either hand to support or to work the foot.

2 It is important to point the fingers of your working hand toward the heel, with the thumb on the sole of the foot providing extra support. Your supporting hand must cup the sole of the foot.

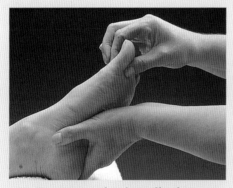

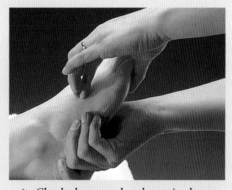

3 To treat people who suffer from congestions in the lymphatic system, it is vital to work the top of the foot as much as the webs between the toes. These reflexes will be sensitive. The reflex between the big and second toes is the throat reflex area and will be particularly sensitive on smokers.

4 Check that your hands are in the correct position – the web between the thumb and index finger of your working hand should touch the web between the toes. Place the middle finger on top of the index finger to achieve greater pressure on the lymphatic reflexes.

The most important lymphatic reflexes are found in the webs between the toes.

5 Work your way back to the webs in small steps. Repeat the procedure on the other foot. The index finger of your working hand is responsible for working the reflexes on the top of the foot.

Use grip 4 to work the webs of the feet in a rotation movement.

The Thoracic Area – the Ball of the Foot

The thoracic area covers the balls of both feet and extends from the base of the toes to the end of the ball. The division between the ball and the arch is clearly demarcated and corresponds to the diaphragm reflex. In the body, the diaphragm separates the thoracic cavity from the abdominal cavity.

Reflexes situated on the balls of the feet are lungs, heart, shoulders, esophagus, bronchi, lymph drainage, thyroid, parathyroid, and thymus.

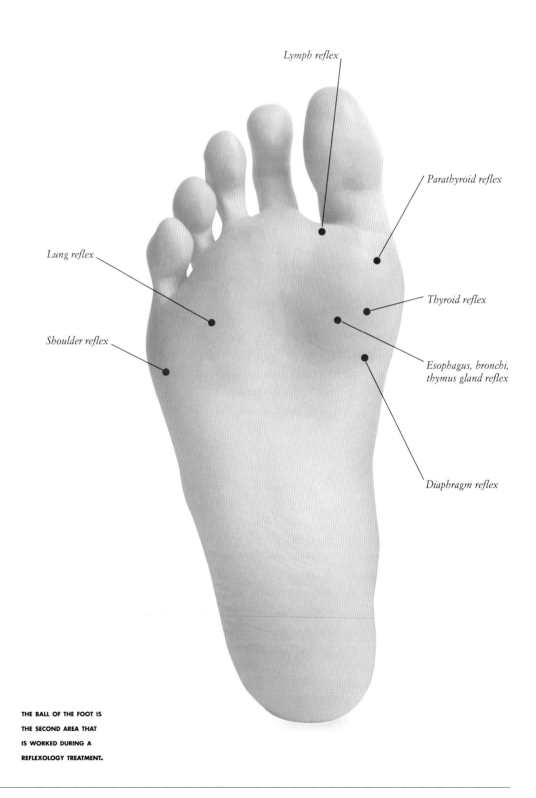

Lymph reflex

Parathyroid reflex

Lung reflex

Thyroid reflex

Shoulder reflex

Esophagus, bronchi, thymus gland reflex

Diaphragm reflex

THE BALL OF THE FOOT IS THE SECOND AREA THAT IS WORKED DURING A REFLEXOLOGY TREATMENT.

BRONCHI, LUNGS, AND HEART

THE BRONCHI AND LUNG REFLEXES ARE SITUATED ON THE BALLS OF BOTH FEET, EXTENDING FROM BELOW THE SECOND TOE
TO JUST BEYOND THE FOURTH TOE. AS THE HEART IS A SINGLE ORGAN FOUND ON THE LEFT SIDE OF THE BODY,
THE HEART REFLEX IS FOUND ON THE LEFT FOOT ONLY.

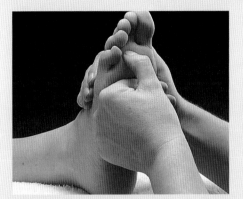

1 Using grip 1 *(see page 142)*, start working on the lung area just below the "shelf" of the chronic eye and ear reflexes *(see page 154)*. Support the foot from the inside using the standard support grip *(see page 132)* with all four fingers and the thumb on the top of the foot. The fist of your working hand provides additional support on the sole of the foot.

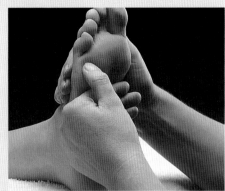

2 You can work moving from left to right, or moving from right to left. You will need to change your supporting hand and your working hand accordingly. In these photographs the left hand is the working hand and the right hand is the supporting hand for working the right foot, this is reversed for working on the left foot.

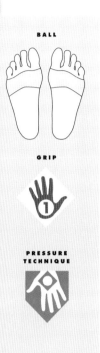

BALL

GRIP

PRESSURE
TECHNIQUE

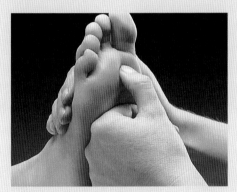

3 You can also work using an up and down technique over this area from the diaphragm to the "shelf." It is important to ensure that the entire area is covered.

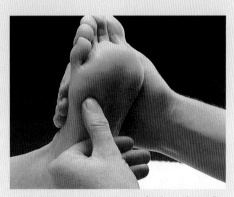

4 Do not work down farther than the lower end of the ball of the foot, which represents the diaphragm reflex.

Work the entire area of the ball of the foot but not lower down than the diaphragm reflex.

5 The heart reflex is lodged in the lung reflex area of the *left* foot, just above the diaphragm line, which is situated on the joint beneath the fourth toe (metatarsal-phalangeal joint).

The heart reflex is found on the left foot only.

THYROID, PARATHYROID, AND NECK

THESE REFLEXES ARE SITUATED ON BOTH FEET, FROM THE BASE OF THE BALL UP TO THE BASE OF THE BIG TOE.
FOR THIS SEQUENCE USE GRIP 5 (SEE PAGE 144). COVER THE ENTIRE AREA THOROUGHLY USING A CIRCULAR MOVEMENT –
AROUND THE BASE OF THE BALL AND UP TO THE BASE OF THE BIG TOE, THE NECK REFLEX.
THE THYROID REFLEX IS OFTEN SENSITIVE, SO PROCEED WITH CARE.

BALL

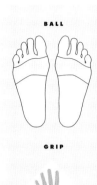

GRIP

PRESSURE
TECHNIQUE

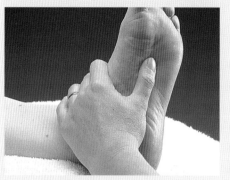

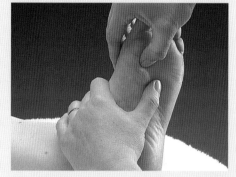

1 If you are working on the left foot, support the foot with your left hand. If you are treating the right foot, support the foot with your right hand. Use the standard support grip *(see page 132)* from the inside, your four fingers on top of the arch and your thumb on the sole.

2 With your working hand use grip 5. Work the reflex area with the tip of your thumb, starting at the base of the ball of the foot.

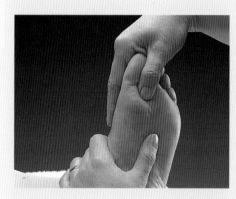

3 Continue to work your way up around the ball of the foot from point to point in small movements.

Support the foot with your four fingers on tip and thumb on the side.

Work the reflexes thoroughly using a circular movement.

Cover the area thoroughly.

4 Work up to your final position at the base of the big toe. This is the neck reflex. Make sure that you have covered the entire area thoroughly.

DIAPHRAGM

THE DIAPHRAGM SEPARATES THE THORACIC CAVITY FROM THE ABDOMINAL CAVITY IN THE BODY.
ITS CORRESPONDING REFLEX SEPARATES THE BALL OF THE FOOT FROM THE ARCH.

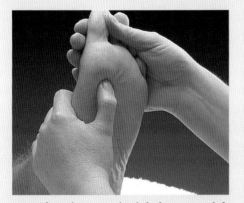

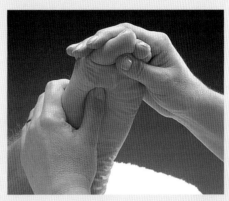

BALL

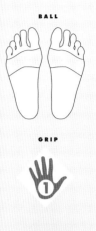

GRIP

PRESSURE TECHNIQUE

1 If working on the left foot, your left hand is the working hand and your right hand is the support hand. Use grip 1 *(see page 142)* with your working hand and the standard support grip *(see page 132)* at the base of the toes with your support hand.

2 With your support hand in the standard support grip, grasp the toes, "lift" them slightly and pull the foot toward you onto your thumb.

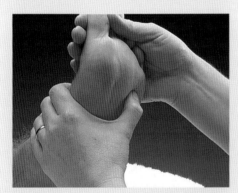

3 With your working hand use the rotating thumb technique *(see page 133)* to work along the diaphragm reflex "line." Your thumb must push up and under the metatarsal bones at a slight angle.

4 Repeat this technique on both feet a couple of times to relax the diaphragm. When working on the right foot, your left hand is the support hand and your right hand is the working hand.

Pull the foot onto your working thumb.

Work along the diaphragm reflex line.

Push the thumb up and under the metatarsal bones.

The Abdominal Area – the Arch of the Foot

All the reflexes related to the digestive system are located in the arch of the foot. This section is often sensitive to pressure. Reflexes here are:

Above the waistline: Right foot – liver, gall bladder, stomach, pancreas, duodenum, kidney, adrenal gland. Left foot – stomach, pancreas, duodenum, spleen, kidney, adrenal gland.

Below the waistline: Right foot – appendix, ileo-cecal valve, ascending colon, transverse colon, small intestine, kidney, ureter, bladder. Left foot – transverse colon, descending colon, sigmoid flexure, rectum, anus, small intestine, kidney, adrenal gland, ureter, bladder.

Since this is a rather complex area, with organs close to and overlapping each other, I have devised a method that I find simplifies the locations of the various organ reflexes.

The arch is clearly visible on the sole of the foot – the raised area that extends from the base of the ball to the beginning of the heel. This is roughly the equivalent of six thumb widths (of the client's thumb) measured horizontally. If the practitioner's thumb is approximately the same size as the client's, the divisions will be perfectly accurate. The first three thumb widths on the inside of the foot cover the reflexes of the stomach, pancreas, and duodenum respectively. These end at the waistline. The three thumb width measures below the waistline cover the large and small intestine reflexes.

BELOW

BY USING A MEASURE OF SIX THUMB WIDTHS, THE PRACTITIONER CAN EASILY IDENTIFY THE REFLEXES ON THE ARCH OF THE FOOT.

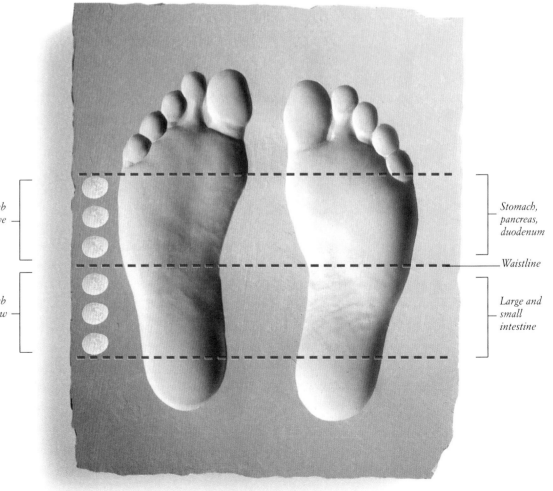

Three thumb widths above waistline.

Three thumb widths below waistline.

Stomach, pancreas, duodenum

Waistline

Large and small intestine

LIVER AND GALL BLADDER

THE LIVER IS THE LARGEST ORGAN IN THE BODY, THUS THE REFLEX COVERS A LARGE AREA. IT IS SITUATED ON THE RIGHT FOOT ONLY. THE GALL BLADDER REFLEX IS CLOSE TO, AND OFTEN EMBEDDED IN, THE LIVER REFLEX – SO CLOSE AS TO BE ALMOST INDISTINGUISHABLE.

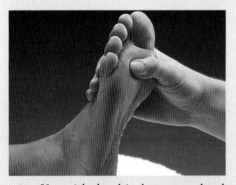

1 Your right hand is the support hand for this technique. Use the standard support grip *(see page 132)* at the base of the toes.

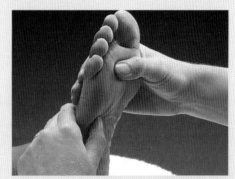

2 Your left hand is the working hand. To locate the liver reflex imagine a triangle below the lung reflex. One side of the triangle is at the outer edge of the foot, the other the diaphragm line. The base cuts diagonally across the arch. Use grip 7 *(see page 145)*.

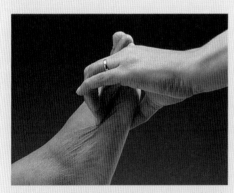

3 The gall bladder reflex is more difficult to locate. Run your finger about 1 in. up toward the ankle between the fourth and fifth toes – in the web between the metatarsals. Here you will find a slight indentation sensitive to pressure. Pinpoint the area directly beneath on the sole of the foot; this is the gall bladder reflex. In some people this is in the middle of the liver reflex.

4 Work the entire liver reflex with your left thumb. If there is sensitivity in this area use the gall bladder exercise.

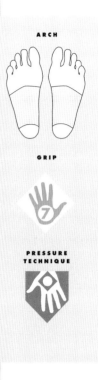

ARCH

GRIP

7

PRESSURE TECHNIQUE

The liver reflex is situated on your right foot only.

The liver reflex covers a large area.

Your left hand is the working hand for this technique.

STOMACH, PANCREAS, DUODENUM, AND SPLEEN

THE STOMACH, PANCREAS, AND DUODENUM REFLEXES ARE FOUND ON BOTH FEET. THE SPLEEN REFLEX IS ON THE LEFT FOOT ONLY. TO LOCATE THE REFLEXES USE THE THUMB MEASURE RULE – THE FIRST THUMB WIDTH PINPOINTS THE STOMACH REFLEX; THE SECOND, THE PANCREAS REFLEX; THE THIRD, THE DUODENUM REFLEX, ENDING ON THE WAISTLINE.

ARCH

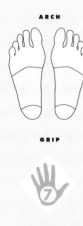

GRIP

PRESSURE
TECHNIQUE

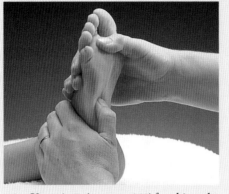

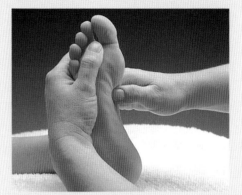

1 Use grip 7 *(see page 145)* for this technique. When working on the right foot, support it with your right hand in the standard support grip *(see page 132)* around the base of the toes and work the outside of the foot with your left hand using the rotating thumb technique *(see page 133)*. This covers the liver reflex *(see previous page)*. Work inward toward the midline of the foot.

2 Now change hands. Support the foot with your left hand and work the inside of the foot with your right hand, again using grip 7. Work three thumb widths through the stomach, pancreas, and duodenum reflexes.

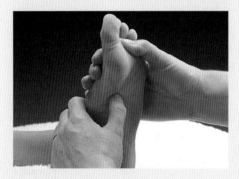

3 Move on to work the left foot. Your right hand is the outside support hand and your left hand works the inside of the foot across the stomach reflex to the halfway mark using grip 7.

Work the outside of the left foot through the spleen reflex.

4 At this point swap hands – support the inside of the foot with your left hand, and work the outside half of the foot with your right hand through the spleen reflex, using grip 7. Finally, change hands again and repeat the same action to work the pancreas and duodenum reflexes on the inside of the left foot below the stomach reflex.

Use grip 7 and the standard support grip for this technique.

SMALL INTESTINE, ILEO-CECAL VALVE, APPENDIX, AND LARGE INTESTINE

IF YOU CONTINUE WITH THE SIX THUMB MEASURES, THE PART OF THE ARCH THAT FALLS UNDER THE FOURTH THUMB IS THE LARGE INTESTINE REFLEX. THE FIFTH AND SIXTH THUMB WIDTHS COVER THE SMALL INTESTINE REFLEX. FOOD IS DIGESTED IN THE SMALL INTESTINE BEFORE IT MOVES INTO THE LARGE INTESTINE, SO IT MAKES SENSE TO STIMULATE THIS AREA FIRST.

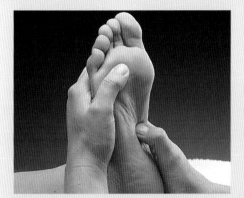

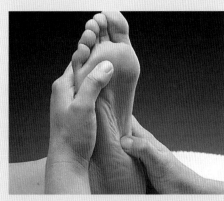

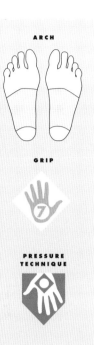

ARCH

GRIP

7

PRESSURE TECHNIQUE

1 Starting with the right foot, support with your left hand from the outside of the foot and work the instep with your right thumb using grip 7 *(see page 145)*. Work the entire square that falls horizontally in the fifth and sixth thumb width areas and vertically to below the fourth toe.

2 There is no need to change hands since the working thumb should be able to stretch far enough across to cover the entire area of this reflex. With the rotating thumb, move up and down or back and forth, depending on preference. The direction of movement is not vital.

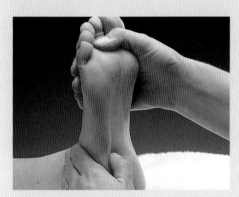

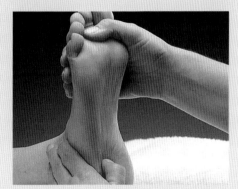

3 The small intestine joins the large intestine at the ileo-cecal valve below the fourth toe in the sixth thumb width. This valve plays an important part in food digestion. If it is not functioning correctly, food particles can enter the large intestine before all the nutrients have been absorbed, or particles from the large intestine may filter back into the small intestine, which could cause infection of the appendix.

4 The appendix reflex is slightly below the ileo-cecal valve reflex. A few seconds pressure can be exerted here with a stationary thumb for extra stimulation. When work on the small intestine area is completed on the right foot, repeat the procedure on the left foot. Now move on to work on the large intestine reflex.

SMALL INTESTINE, ILEO-CECAL VALVE, APPENDIX, AND LARGE INTESTINE CONTINUED

THE LARGE INTESTINE REFLEX IS WORKED ON IN THE SAME DIRECTIONS AS IT FUNCTIONS IN THE BODY – UP THE ASCENDING COLON, ACROSS THE TRANSVERSE COLON AND DOWN THE DESCENDING COLON TO THE RECTUM. BECAUSE FOOD PARTICLES CAN EASILY BECOME LODGED IN THE CORNERS (FLEXURES), THESE AREAS MUST BE WORKED FIRMLY TO STIMULATE THE FLOW.

ARCH

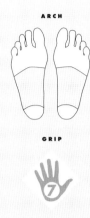

GRIP

PRESSURE TECHNIQUE

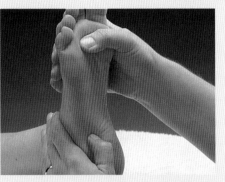

5 Still using grip 7, start on the right foot and the ileo-cecal valve/appendix reflex. Your left hand works on the outside of the foot, your right hand supports from the instep at the base of the toes.

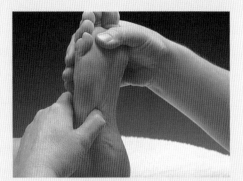

6 Work the rotating thumb up to the liver reflex (hepatic flexure), turn into the transverse colon. Work with your left hand to the halfway mark, then change to work with your right hand and complete the other half of the foot.

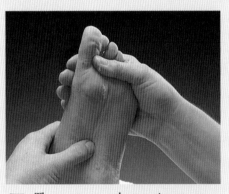

7 The transverse colon continues over to the left foot; support with your right hand from the outside of the foot and work the inside of the foot with your left hand, until you reach the center of the foot.

Support from the inside at the back of the toes.

Apply extra pressure at the flexures.

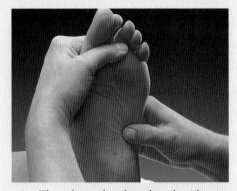

8 Then change hands and work with your right hand on the outside of the foot and support with your left hand from the inside of the foot to complete the transverse colon reflex area. Turn below the spleen (splenic flexure) and work down the side of the foot along the descending colon.

9 Curve into the sigmoid colon and continue to the rectum/anus reflex. Remember to apply extra pressure at the flexures since congestion frequently occurs in these areas. Change working hands whenever necessary for your own comfort.

ONCE THIS SECTION IS COMPLETE, THE ENTIRE DIGESTIVE SYSTEM HAS BEEN STIMULATED.

KIDNEYS AND ADRENALS

THE KIDNEYS ARE PAIRED ORGANS, SO REFLEXES ARE FOUND ON BOTH FEET. THE ADRENAL GLAND REFLEXES ARE DIRECTLY ABOVE THE KIDNEY REFLEXES SO ARE WORKED SIMULTANEOUSLY WITH THE KIDNEYS. USE GRIP 7 (SEE PAGE 145). ALWAYS WORK WITH YOUR INSIDE HAND (LEFT FOR THE LEFT FOOT, RIGHT FOR THE RIGHT FOOT) AND SUPPORT WITH YOUR OUTSIDE HAND (RIGHT FOR THE LEFT FOOT, LEFT FOR THE RIGHT FOOT) USING THE STANDARD SUPPORT GRIP (SEE PAGE 132).

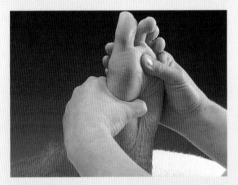
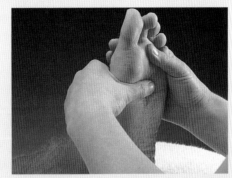
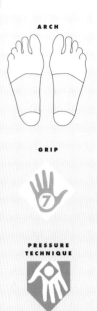

ARCH

GRIP

PRESSURE TECHNIQUE

1 The kidney and adrenal reflexes are worked using grip 7 (see page 145).

2 The reflexes are found approximately one thumb measure below the solar plexus reflex. This is in the central indentation on the diaphragm line dividing the ball of the foot from the arch.

3 Go in with the thumb of your working hand, rotate and lift.

Support the foot using the standard support grip.

Use the rotating thumb technique.

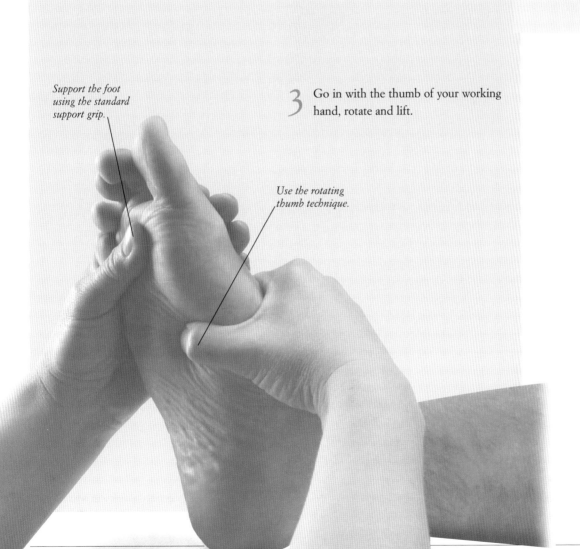

URETERS AND BLADDER

THE TECHNIQUE DESCRIBED HERE IS SPECIFICALLY FOR WORKING THE URETER AND BLADDER REFLEXES.
THE URETER REFLEX IS OFTEN "MAPPED" ON THE FOOT, AS A CURVED LINE DESCENDING ACROSS THE ARCH TOWARD
THE BLADDER REFLEX UNDER THE INNER ANKLE BONE.

ARCH

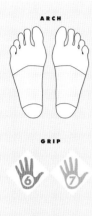

GRIP

PRESSURE
TECHNIQUE

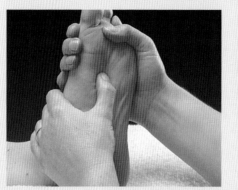

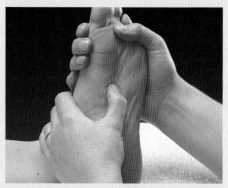

1 Work the ureter reflex using grip 7 *(see page 145)*. Work the inside of the foot with your inside hand and support with your outside hand. Hold the foot using the standard support grip *(see page 132)* at the base of the toes.

2 Continue to work down the ureter reflex toward the bladder reflex, exerting pressure with the rotating thumb.

3 The bladder reflex is roughly the size of a large coin. The whole area should be carefully worked on with the rotating thumb; this area is often puffy, particularly if there is a bladder imbalance.

4 When you reach the bladder reflex, change to grip 6. Support the foot with the standard support grip and cup the foot in the palm of your working hand, leaving the thumb free to work the reflex.

The bladder reflex should be worked on carefully, particularly if the area is puffy.

Change to grip 6 when you reach the bladder reflex.

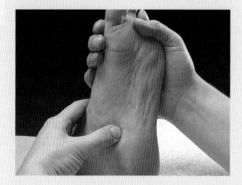

The Pelvic Area – the Heel of the Foot

Because the heel is usually quite tough, the pelvic area is the toughest to work on. The skin is often hard and darker than the rest of the foot because of the fact that the heel bears the brunt of the body weight when walking. As a result, few people feel any pain in this area. This does not detract from the fact that it is an important area to work well, and you may need to apply more pressure to stimulate the reflexes effectively. Many people suffer from congestions in the pelvic area and this may be aggravated by the presence of numerous meridians in the heel.

PELVIS AND SCIATIC NERVE

THESE REFLEXES CAN BE STIMULATED USING THE KNEAD OR ROTATING THUMB TECHNIQUE.

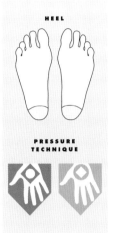

HEEL

PRESSURE TECHNIQUE

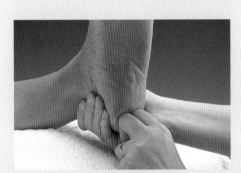

1 Choose whichever hand feels most comfortable to work with. Support the foot by cupping the back of the ankle in the palm of your supporting hand. Keep the heel area free.

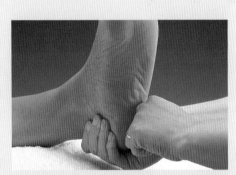

2 Make a fist with your working hand. Execute the knead technique (*see page 135*), using the knuckles of the second joint of the fingers to "knead" the heel – a similar technique to kneading bread.

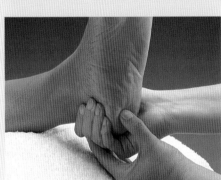

3 If the client has a very soft heel, a more gentle method of stimulation would be to use the rotating thumb technique (*see page 133*), exerting less pressure.

Either with your knuckles or using the rotating thumb technique, work the pelvic area of the heel well.

You can choose which hand to work with and which to provide support but ensure that the foot is held securely.

4 The sciatic reflex and nerve run horizontally across the heel so will automatically be stimulated as you work the pelvic area of the heel.

The Reproductive Area – the Ankle

All the reproductive organ reflexes are situated around the ankle area. These are ovaries, testes, uterus, prostate, Fallopian tubes, and vas deferens.

UTERUS, PROSTATE, OVARIES AND TESTES

WHEN WORKING ON THE LEFT FOOT, SUPPORT IT WITH YOUR RIGHT HAND AND USE YOUR LEFT HAND TO WORK THE INNER REFLEXES. TO WORK THE OUTER REFLEXES, SUPPORT THE FOOT WITH YOUR LEFT HAND AND WORK WITH YOUR RIGHT HAND. WHEN WORKING ON THE RIGHT FOOT, SUPPORT IT WITH YOUR LEFT HAND AND USE YOUR RIGHT HAND. TO WORK THE OUTER REFLEXES, SUPPORT THE FOOT WITH YOUR RIGHT HAND AND WORK WITH YOUR LEFT.

ANKLE

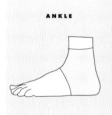

GRIP

PRESSURE TECHNIQUE

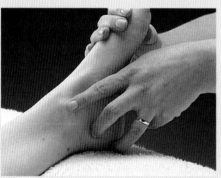

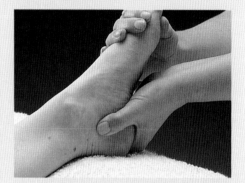

1 The uterus and prostate reflexes are located on the inner foot below the ankle bone. To pinpoint the exact area place the tip of the index finger on the ankle bone and the tip of the ring finger on the back corner of the heel. With the middle finger, establish an exact midpoint in a straight line.

3 To work the uterus/prostate area, use grip 6 *(see page 144)*, as with the bladder. Cup your working hand at the back of the ankle. Hold the foot with your support hand using the standard support grip *(see page 132)* close to the toes. The area to cover is approximately the size of a large coin. Repeat the procedure on both feet.

2 The ovaries/testes reflexes are in the same area, but below the outside ankle bone. Locate the reflexes with the same technique described for the uterus/prostate.

Working the area below the outside of the ankle bone stimulates the ovaries/testes reflexes.

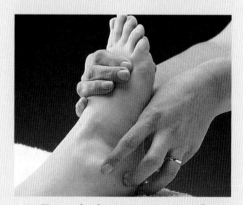

4 To work the ovaries/testes reflexes, again use grip 6. Work below the outside of the ankle bone, covering the entire area.

FALLOPIAN TUBES AND VAS DEFERENS

THIS TECHNIQUE WORKS THE FALLOPIAN TUBE REFLEX IN FEMALES AND VAS DEFERENS REFLEX IN MALES, WHICH RUN FROM THE INNER ANKLE BONE ALONG THE TOP OF THE FOOT AT THE BASE OF THE ANKLE TO THE OUTER ANKLE BONE. STEPS 1 AND 2 SHOW THE STARTING POINT ON THE INNER AND OUTER ANKLE BONE. STEP 3 IS PERFORMED USING FINGER TECHNIQUE 2 (SEE PAGE 134). STEP 4 PROVIDES AN ALTERNATIVE FOR STEPS 1 AND 2.

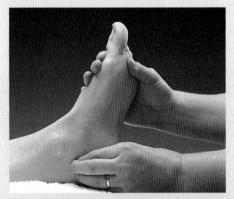

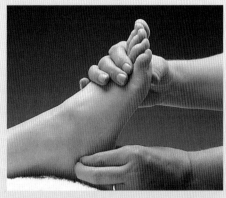

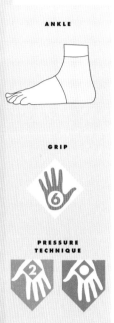

ANKLE

GRIP

PRESSURE
TECHNIQUE

1 The reflex for the Fallopian tube or vas deferens starts at the base of the inner ankle bone.

2 The Fallopian tube or vas deferens reflex runs right over the top of the foot to the outer ankle.

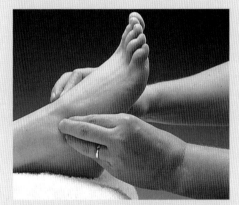

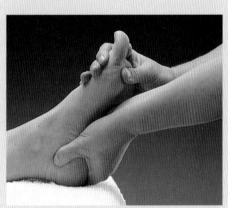

3 Now use finger technique 2 (see page 134) and move along the top of the foot from the base of the ankle bone until both hands meet.

4 An alternative technique for working the Fallopian tube or vas deferens reflex is to use grip 6, with the palm of your working hand doubling as additional support on the heel and sole of the foot. Work the rotating thumb from the uterus/prostate reflex to the ovaries/testes reflex.

The Spine – the Inner Foot

The spine reflex runs the length of the inside of the foot. Treating this reflex will activate blood flow to the spine, loosen vertebrae and muscles in this area, and have a stimulating effect on the entire body by invigorating activity of the nerve impulses. As the spine represents the midline of the body, the reflex is found in the same area on both feet. The reflex area on each foot corresponds with half the spine. It is vital to work this area thoroughly, and often "tight" areas will be found.

SPINE

THE SPINAL TWIST IS USED AT THE BEGINNING OF THIS SEQUENCE FOR RELAXATION.

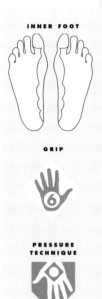

INNER FOOT

GRIP

PRESSURE TECHNIQUE

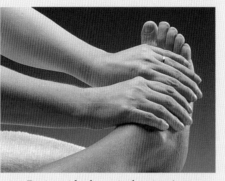

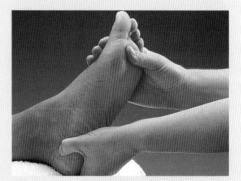

1 Begin with the spinal twist (see page 139). Grasp the foot with both hands on the inside of the instep. The hand closest to the ankle provides support. Your working hand twists backward and forward. Move your hands along the foot toward the toes, and work the foot again. Repeat this movement until the entire length of the foot has been covered.

2 To work the lumber reflex, use grip 6 (see page 144), cupping the foot in the palm of your working hand. Keep the thumb free to work the reflex using the rotating thumb technique. On the left foot, your right hand is the supporting hand using the standard support grip (see page 132) at the base of the toes. Your left hand is then your working hand.

3 Start at the tip of the heel and work up the spine to the toes. Use the rotating thumb effectively, loosening each vertebrae. If you bend the toes toward you slightly with your support hand, you can see the spine reflex quite clearly. Work along the bony structure on the instep. Do not work directly on the bone, but slightly under it, using the bone as your guideline.

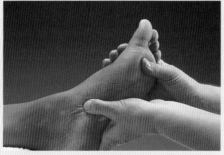

Pay special attention to the base of the big toe.

The spine reflex runs the length of the inside of the foot.

Use the bony structure on the instep of the foot as a guidance to the spine reflex.

4 Pay special attention to the base of the big toe because these are the reflexes of the seven cervical vertebrae.

Outer Body – the Outer Foot

The technique employed here is excellent for treating conditions affecting the knee, hip, elbow, or shoulder. The outer body reflexes run the length of the outside of each foot, from the tip of the heel to the tip of the fifth (little) toe. The shoulder reflex is found at the base of the little toe.

KNEE, HIP, ELBOW, AND SHOULDER

THIS SEQUENCE ALSO INCLUDES WORK ON THE GALL BLADDER MERIDIANS.

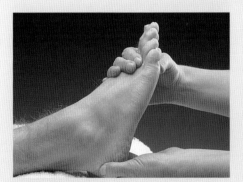

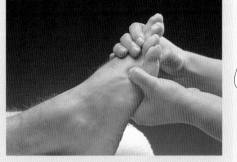

OUTER FOOT

GRIP

6

PRESSURE
TECHNIQUE

1 Use grip 6 as with the spinal reflex, but with opposite hands. If you are working on the right foot, support the top of the foot with your right hand and work with your left. If you are working on the left foot, support the top of the foot with your left hand and work with your right. Begin at the tip of the heel and work toward the toes.

2 Continue to move along the side of the foot until you are in line with the fourth toe. This is the gall bladder meridian, which runs through the hip region. This area may be puffy, which could indicate hip weakness or posture problems associated with the lower back.

3 Now move to the outer edge of the foot to locate the shoulder reflex, working with the rotating thumb technique.

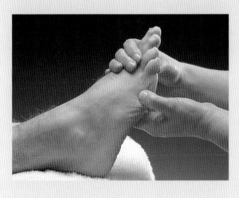

Work along the reflex toward the toes.

The outer body reflexes run from the tip of the outer heel to the outer tip of the little toe.

4 Work from the area at the base of the little toe that corresponds to the outside of the shoulder in line to the tip of the little toe.

Circulation and Breasts – the Top of the Foot

BREASTS AND CIRCULATION

THE REFLEXES FOR THE BREASTS AND CIRCULATION ARE SITUATED ON THE TOPS OF BOTH FEET. THIS TECHNIQUE IS PART
OF THE WINDING DOWN STAGE OF THE TREATMENT SO CREAM OR OIL CAN BE APPLIED TO FACILITATE MOVEMENT
AND VARIOUS RELAXING MASSAGE TECHNIQUES CAN BE USED. THE LAST THREE TECHNIQUES SHOULD GLIDE INTO
EACH OTHER AS THE FINAL TREATMENT STAGE.

TOPS

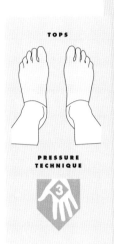

**PRESSURE
TECHNIQUE**

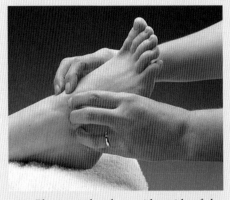

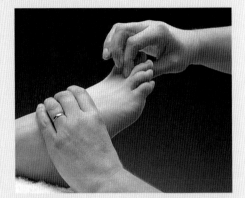

1 Place your hands on either side of the foot with the thumbs on the sole acting as support, and the fingers on the top of the foot. Using finger technique 3 *(see page 134)*, massage down the foot slowly and gently, making sure the technique is relaxing for the client. Repeat the procedure on both feet.

2 To finish this treatment, support the foot with one hand on the arch while applying extra pressure to the special circulation points in the webs between the second and third toes with your other hand.

KIDNEY AND BLADDER MERIDIANS

THE KIDNEY MERIDIAN RUNS UP THE BACK OF THE ANKLE ALONG THE ACHILLES TENDON. STIMULATING THIS SECTION IS
INCORPORATED INTO THE MASSAGE BEGUN IN THE PREVIOUS MOVEMENT.

**PRESSURE
TECHNIQUE**

1 Support the ankle in whichever hand feels most comfortable. Slide the fingers of your other hand back up the ankle along the Achilles tendon. You can do this either on the inside or on the outside of the leg, again whichever feels most comfortable.

*Take care when using
this technique since
the area worked on
may be sensitive.*

*Apply pressure to this
meridian by gently pinching
the Achilles tendon.*

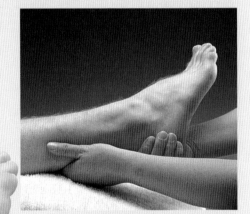

2 Apply the pinch technique *(see page 135)* by gently pinching the Achilles tendon at the back of the heel with your working hand as it moves up and down the tendon. This area may be extremely sensitive so proceed with care.

SOLAR PLEXUS DEEP BREATHING

THE SOLAR PLEXUS IS REFERRED TO AS THE "NERVE SWITCHBOARD" OF THE BODY AND IS THE MAIN STRESS STORAGE AREA. WORKING ON THIS AREA WILL ALWAYS INDUCE RELAXATION AND CAN BE USED AT ANY POINT DURING THE TREATMENT. THE TECHNIQUE TO USE IS DESCRIBED IN "RELAXATION TECHNIQUES" (SEE PAGE 141). IT IS ALWAYS USED TO ROUND OFF A TREATMENT. ASK THE CLIENT TO TAKE DEEP BREATHS (ABOUT THREE) AND APPLY PRESSURE TO THE SOLAR PLEXUS REFLEXES.

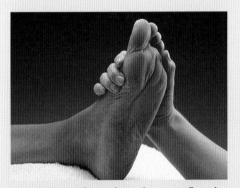

1 Locate the solar plexus reflex by squeezing the sides of the foot together to form a depression. The reflex will be found where this line meets the diaphragm under the ball of the foot.

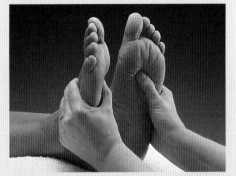

2 Gripping the feet, place your left thumb on the solar plexus reflex on the right foot, and your right thumb on the reflex of the left foot.

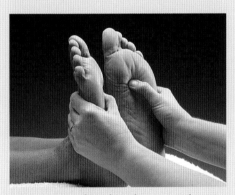

3 As your client breathes in, apply pressure to the reflexes. As the client breathes out, release the pressure.

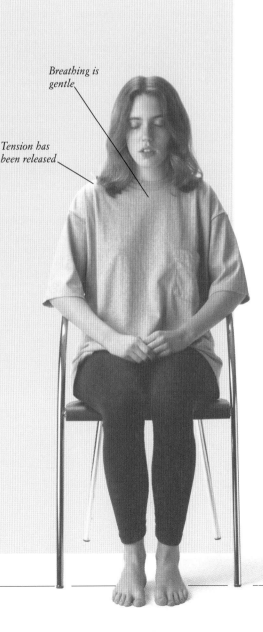

Breathing is gentle

Tension has been released

RIGHT
Following treatment, the client should sit quietly and relax for a few minutes.

The VacuFlex Reflexology System

The VacuFlex Reflexology System evolved from an idea I first came upon in Denmark. Over a period of 12 years, I have developed and systemized this approach to reflexology in order to modernize the practice.

The full VacuFlex treatment is a two-phase treatment that combines the stimulation of the foot reflexes with rebalancing of the meridians. This system is often referred to as the "boot" system because of the large spacesuit-like felt boots used on the feet. The VacuFlex system combines three alternative therapies – reflexology, acupressure, and cupping. This combination has proved to be effective in relieving problems otherwise difficult to combat, such as back problems, strokes, circulation problems, and arthritis.

Vacuum therapy is acknowledged as an ancient treatment, having been practiced since primitive times when animal horns were used as cups. Cups made from burned clay were discovered in ancient Mesopotamia. In Greece these cups were made of bronze, while other examples have been found constructed of brass, porcelain, and glass. The VacuFlex cups, referred to as "pads," are made of silicone.

Needles, lasers, finger pressure, or suction pads placed on specific meridian points stimulate relaxed nerves, which transmit electrical impulses to the spinal cord and brain. The suction pressure increases the flow of blood and oxygen to congested areas, causing toxic stagnation to disperse. The pressure also encourages tissue and muscle regeneration by stimulating blood supply and nutrients to the affected areas.

The VacuFlex boots come in two sizes, adults and children. The plastic covered boots, which are connected to a vacuum pump, are placed on the feet. Air is suctioned from the boots to create a uniform pressure over the entire foot, which stimulates all the reflexes. This provides a full

ABOVE
In VacuFlex treatment a vacuum is created inside felt boots resulting in a uniform pressure over the foot stimulating all the reflexes.

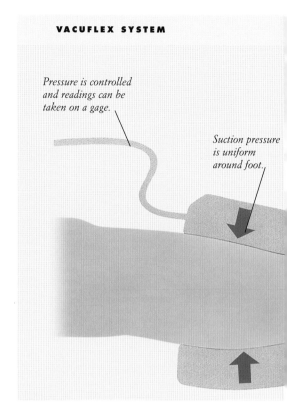

VACUFLEX SYSTEM

Pressure is controlled and readings can be taken on a gage.

Suction pressure is uniform around foot.

reflexology treatment in just five minutes. The pressure can be controlled, and a reading is possible on the pressure gage.

The pressure from the boots leaves a map of colors on the feet for approximately 15 seconds. These colors relate to

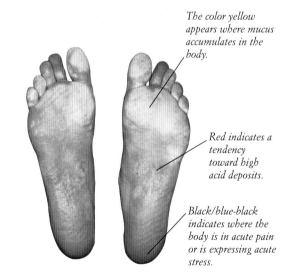

The color yellow appears where mucus accumulates in the body.

Red indicates a tendency toward high acid deposits.

Black/blue-black indicates where the body is in acute pain or is expressing acute stress.

ABOVE
When boots are removed a map of colors can be seen on the foot for 15–30 seconds. These relate to the reflexes that are congested at that precise moment. White (not shown here), indicates a chronic or long-term condition.

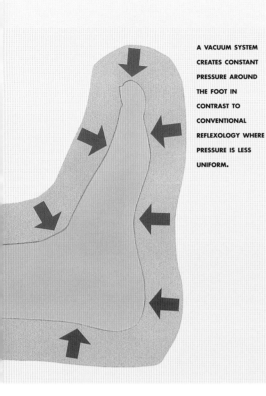

A VACUUM SYSTEM CREATES CONSTANT PRESSURE AROUND THE FOOT IN CONTRAST TO CONVENTIONAL REFLEXOLOGY WHERE PRESSURE IS LESS UNIFORM.

The solar plexus, known as the abdominal brain because it contains so many nerves and nerve networks, is also stimulated by the boots during the first stage of treatment with the result that spasms and cramps cannot occur. It is for this reason that the system was found particularly beneficial in its original development to help a spastic epileptic child who had suffered cramps and spasms during conventional reflexology treatment.

It is often assumed that the pressure exerted by the boots is stronger than the thumb pressure techniques. This is not so. A test conducted by an engineer proved that the pressure applied using the central portion of the tip of the thumb exerts 5.29 times more pressure than the lowest scale of the VacuFlex System, which ranges from 40 to 80 kilopascals. The difference is that the boots apply uniform, constant pressure for a period of five minutes, while the thumb pressure is not uniform or constant.

the reflexes that would have been sore or sensitive during a manual massage. The colors are blue, red, yellow, and white, depending on the severity of the problem. They change from treatment to treatment in accordance with the healing process.

Some people are wary of the system because they feel that the use of mechanical equipment diminishes the interaction between client and practitioner. This is not necessarily so. The vital energy exchange is still apparent since the movement of the pads is physical. Also, the treatment should always be completed with hand-executed relaxation techniques described earlier in this book. People generally find the boot less painful than hand massage, and children can be treated comfortably with this system. The thoroughness of the VacuFlex system ensures that the client always receives a complete and effective treatment irrespective of the practitioner's accuracy.

This system has proved successful in alleviating a wide range of disorders. Research studies into back pain, for example, indicate a high level of efficacy. (See Carol Bosiger's study for detailed case histories, published in 1989 in *The Journal of Alternative and Complementary Medicine*.)

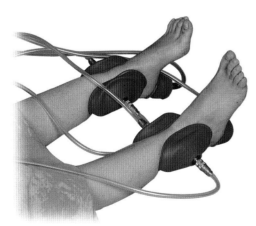

ABOVE
The second stage of the treatment involves stimulating some of the strategic acupuncture points along the meridians of the arms and legs. This is applied with suction pads operated by the same vacuum system as the boots.

13. FOOTCARE

*I*n the average 70-year lifespan, our feet cover about 70,000 miles. This is the equivalent of 2.5 times around the world and averages 1,000 miles a year.[1] This is extremely impressive; so considering how much our feet do for us, how much do we do for them in return? Very little. In the Western world, millions of people are treated annually for foot problems and deformities. Despite these distressing statistics, little attention is afforded to correct footcare. A health-conscious person may pay a great deal of attention to diet, avoiding the hazards of food additives, smoking, and other forms of pollution, but is often completely unaware of the health damage caused by ill-fitting shoes.

ABOVE
This baby's foot is perfectly formed and unblemished, and is yet to have life's experiences impressed on it.

ABOVE
Our feet have to walk approximately 70,000 miles in our lifetime – two and a half times around the equator.

Foot disorders disrupt our center of gravity and can cause knee, leg, and calf pain as well as severe backache and knee instability. As meridians and reflexes are also affected, problems can arise in corresponding parts of the body.

Most foot disorders can be avoided and corrected with correct foot and health care. A little time and attention will not only keep your feet looking good but will have further health benefits. Having practiced the techniques, you are now in a position to appreciate how every part of the foot represents a part of the body, so the relevance of treating the feet with care and kindness is obvious.

ABOVE
Fashion demands that we wear unsuitable footwear. High-heeled shoes throw the body's weight onto the ball of the foot in contrast to low-heeled forms of footwear.

Hammertoe forced out of alignment by bunion.

A callus develops when shoes rub on sensitive skin.

Cramped toes caused by tight-fitting shoes

Rough skin on tops of feet due to neglect.

Swollen ankles are often the result of pressure from excess weight.

LEFT
Years of constraint in ill-fitting shoes have cramped and rubbed this adult's toes.

1 – MICHELLE ARNOT "FOOT NOTES" P3

HYGIENE

Good hygiene is of primary importance. Foot hygiene focuses on washing the feet thoroughly every day to remove dead skin and eliminate bacteria.

The average foot gives off about half a cup of moisture a day. The skin becomes soft and soggy as a result of the moisture, making it easier for friction to cause blisters, for chemicals to leach from shoes and cause contact dermatitis, and for athlete's foot and other forms of fungal infection to take hold.

The most common problem from all that moisture is bromhidrosis – a scientific term for smelly feet. This occurs because the foot's warmth and sweat provide choice growing conditions for bacteria. Good foot hygiene will help combat this by reducing perspiration. Perspiration can also be reduced by paying special attention to the type of footwear you use.

Feet should also be kept warm and comfortable at all times. Changes in foot temperature can exacerbate health problems. People living in a warm subtropical climate, for example, may find that sinus problems, runny noses, chest problems, and bladder weakness are common among children. Due to the high outdoor temperatures, air conditioning is common in this climate. Thus children are constantly moving between the hot outdoor and cool indoors, usually barefoot. A rapid drop in foot temperature will have an adverse effect on the reflexes and meridians, and thereby the related organs.

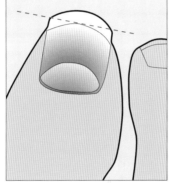

ABOVE
Always trim your nails straight across.

BASIC FOOTCARE HINTS

★ Wash your feet carefully and dry thoroughly, especially between the toes.

★ Allow your feet to "air out." Don't keep them locked up in shoes all the time.

★ Trim your toenails straight across.

★ Use creams to keep the skin supple and powders on your feet to absorb extra moisture and prevent infection and odor.

★ Regular pedicures are beneficial.

★ Regular washing and careful drying will help to prevent cracks from developing.

★ A pumice stone and creams will help soften hardened areas.

★ Problems such as corns, plantar warts, and athlete's foot should be attended to, and a chiropodist consulted for persistent problems.

Short, well-cut toenails.

Dry thoroughly between the toes to reduce the risk of athlete's foot.

ABOVE
Wash the feet and dry thoroughly, concentrating on the areas between the toes.

ABOVE
Rub any areas of hard or dry skin firmly but gently with a pumice stone to soften and remove any flakes.

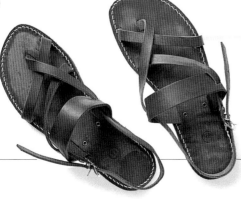

LEFT
Flat, leather sandals are the best form of footwear for your feet. Air can circulate, preventing pockets of moisture from getting trapped between the toes.

CASE STUDY

A young male client suffered constant sinus and chest problems, and asthma attacks. He responded well to reflexology treatments, but there was a constant recurrence of asthma attacks and often a slight cold. I checked his daily routine.

On rising in the morning he would go straight from his warm bed into the yard (onto the cool, dew-covered grass) to let out the dogs and collect his newspaper. He would then go back indoors for a shower and walk around barefoot on tiled floors.

The rapid variations in foot temperature were having an adverse effect on his entire body, causing this propensity to colds and asthma.

I recommended that he wear shoes rather than go barefoot to keep his foot temperature constant, and his condition improved tremendously.

Temperature going up in warm bed.

Temperature going down sharply from wet grass.

Temperature up again in hot shower.

Temperature down again on cold tiles.

Collecting newspaper from cold outdoors lowers body temperature.

Hot shower raises body temperature.

Hot drink raises body temperature.

Walking barefoot on cold floor lowers body temperature.

RAPID CHANGES OF THE PATIENT'S BODY TEMPERATURE ADVERSELY AFFECTED HIS RESPONSE TO REFLEXOLOGY TREATMENT.

RIGHT
If you prefer being barefoot you should make sure the temperature is constant – rapid variations can lead to colds and asthma.

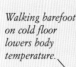

Shoes, Socks, and Pantyhose

Most adults have abused their feet, mainly by wearing ill-fitting shoes. There are no shoes on the market that conform to the outline of the human foot – this is obvious if you just place your shoe beside your foot and compare the shape. Another factor is that no-one has two identical feet – one foot is always slightly larger than the other. High-heeled shoes are probably the worst culprits since they affect the body weight, balance and, thereby, the spine. Synthetic shoes should also be avoided since they do not ventilate, thus increasing the risk of fungal infection. Rubber and plastic shoes will also stifle the feet. Low-heeled, lightweight, leather or natural fiber shoes are the best. So choose your shoes carefully; your health depends on it.[2]

Socks and stockings made of synthetic material should also be avoided, since they increase the likelihood of sweating. Choose 100 percent cotton or wool rather than nylon or mixtures of fibers.

Wide fitting across foot.

Leather

Firm support at sides and top

Low heels *Solid soles*

ABOVE
Natural fiber socks – 100 percent wool or cotton – are best for healthy feet.

ABOVE
Choose wide fitting leather shoes with low heels and good support to protect your feet.

Lavender

BELOW
The healing properties of herbs effectively penetrate the skin in a herbal foot bath.

Feet Treats

FOOT BATHS

Famous herbalist and healer Maurice Messegue recommended herbal foot baths as an essential part of his treatment. He believed treatment by osmosis to be most effective since the main healing ingredients rapidly penetrate the skin and sometimes reach the affected areas faster than if the same ingredients are taken internally. He chose foot and hand baths over hip and full baths since they are easy to prepare and because the hands and feet are the most receptive parts of the body.

Baths can be prepared with dried herbs or aromatherapy oils infused in boiling water. Foot baths should be taken as hot as possible (but not boiling), first thing in the morning on an empty stomach, and should not last for more than eight minutes.

Sweet Marjoram

ABOVE
Lavender and Sweet Marjoram are effective herbs for use in foot baths.

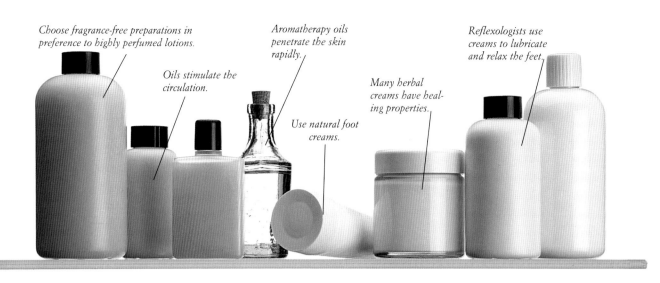

Choose fragrance-free preparations in preference to highly perfumed lotions.

Oils stimulate the circulation.

Aromatherapy oils penetrate the skin rapidly.

Use natural foot creams.

Many herbal creams have healing properties.

Reflexologists use creams to lubricate and relax the feet.

ABOVE
Pamper your feet with generous applications of creams and oils, both during and between treatments.

CREAMS AND OILS

A therapist may apply herbal ointment or oil to stimulate circulation and relax the client at the end of a treatment. It is a good idea to pamper your feet like this at regular intervals – either after a self-treatment or merely to relax and revitalize your feet. There are numerous foot creams on the market, but it is preferable to use something natural and herbal like aromatherapy oils or herbal creams since they contain beneficial healing properties.

Chemical foot sprays should be avoided. They clog the pores and stop the feet from ridding themselves and the body of excretions from the sweat glands. It is not wise to suppress the ability of the body to perspire through the feet. Excessive sweating is an indication of imbalance and should not be ignored.

OTHER FOOT AIDS

There are numerous "foot aids" available on the market today: reflexology mats; wood or plastic rollers; brushes and electrically operated gadgets; and many types of balls. These help tone and relax the foot and increase lymphatic drainage and circulation but should be used in moderation to prevent overstimulation. They are effective for health maintenance, but not for treating specific problems.

When using any of the "roller" type aids, roll them in a uniform way with an even, light pressure over the entire foot – bottom and sides. No special emphasis need be placed on any particular reflexes. Apply this rolling therapy every day for approximately ten minutes per foot.

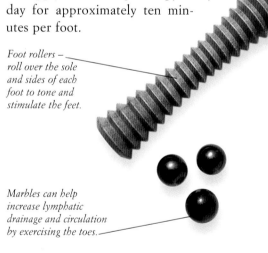

Foot rollers – roll over the sole and sides of each foot to tone and stimulate the feet.

Marbles can help increase lymphatic drainage and circulation by exercising the toes.

ABOVE
Exercise and stimulate the foot by regular use of rollers and balls.

ABOVE
*Walking barefoot
is the best form of
exercise for your
feet.*

EXERCISE

Correct and regular foot exercise will not only keep the feet in good shape but can also combat deformities. Specific exercises are often prescribed by physiotherapists for chronic foot disorders, with excellent results.

There are some simple, easy exercises that can be done at home or the office, which will be beneficial to the feet and should be practiced whenever the opportunity arises.

FOOT EXERCISES

1 Rotate the foot to limber it up.

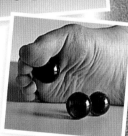

2 To tone up ligaments and tendons, pick up marbles with the toes.

3 To strengthen the arches, stand with your feet flat on the floor and curl the toes under.

Walking is one of the best and simplest forms of exercise – walk barefoot as often as possible to allow your feet to recover from the confinement of shoes. Barefooted people are less likely to develop foot deformities. A natural foot massage is by far the best – and probably more effective than any gadget. A barefoot walk on the beach, grass, or bare earth brings the feet into contact with the earth, and the energies that flow through it to provide a revitalizing, energizing, and natural massage.

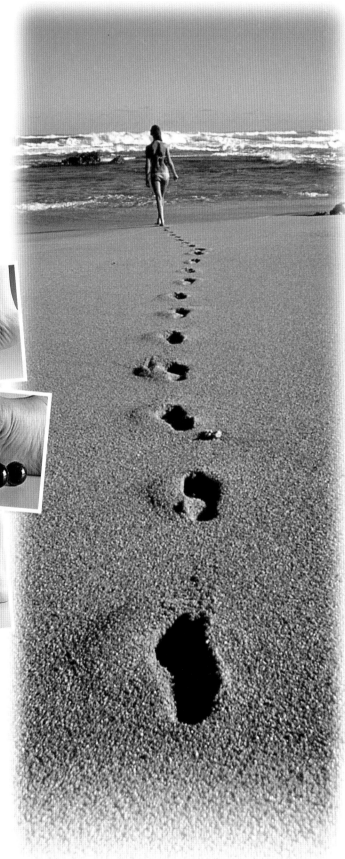

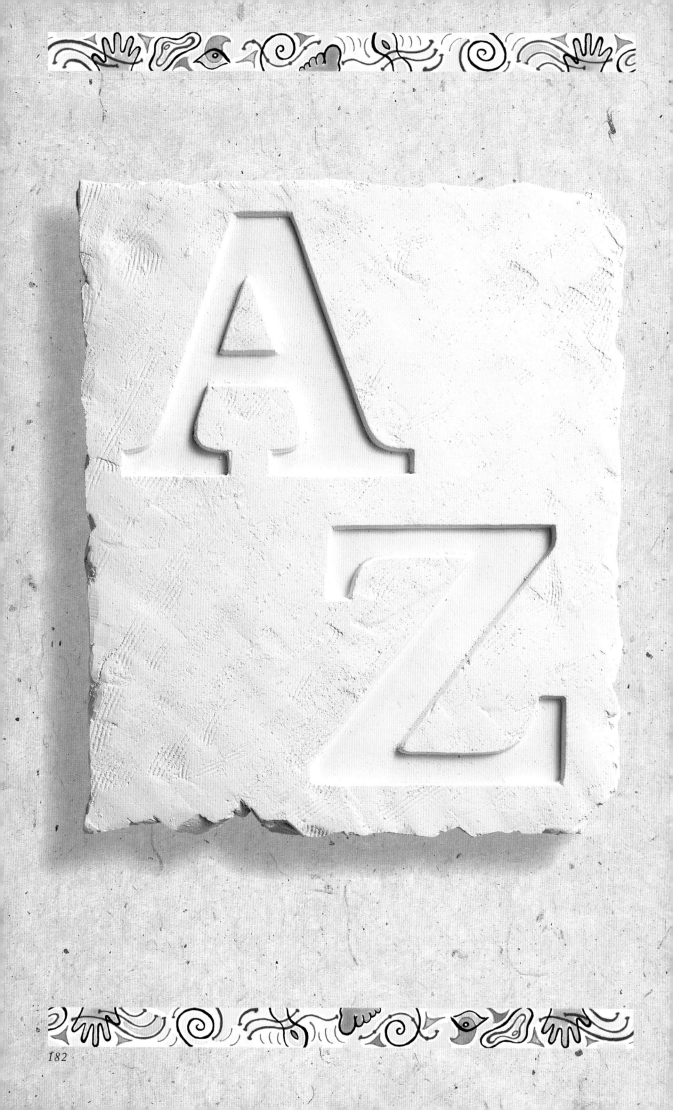

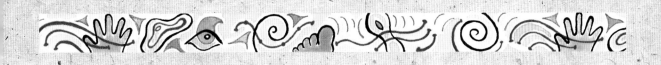

PART FOUR

REFERENCE
SECTION

GLOSSARY

ABDOMINAL pertaining to the abdomen, the part of the body lying between chest and pelvis

ACHILLES' TENDON the attachment of the soleus and gastrocnemius muscles of the calf of the leg to the heel bone

ACNE common skin disorder usually caused by hormone imbalance (especially during adolescence)

ACUPRESSURE works on the same basic principle as acupuncture, but the ch'i is worked on by pressure and massage instead of needles

ACUPUNCTURE Chinese healing therapy designed to rebalance or unblock the flow of energy within the body. Needles are used at certain points on the body, which correspond to points on the meridians along which the energy is thought to flow; see also acupuncture points; meridians

ADRENAL GLAND a two-part gland situated just above each kidney

ADRENALIN substance secreted by part of the adrenal gland that increases the heart rate in response to stress

ADRENOCORTICAL pertaining to the adrenal cortex, the outer part of the ductless adrenal glands

ANESTHETIC loss of feeling or sensation; substance that causes such a loss

ANGINA PECTORIS severe pain in the lower chest, usually on the left side

ANOREXIA NERVOSA psychological problem causing extreme loss of appetite and drastic weight loss

ANTIALLERGIC substance that reduces allergic reactions

ANTIINFLAMMATORY substance that alleviates inflammation

APPENDIX a worm-shaped projection from between the junction of the small intestine and the cecum; it no longer plays any function in the human digestive process

ARTHRITIS painful inflammation of joint tissues

ASTHMA spasm of the bronchi in the lungs, narrowing the airwaves

ATHLETE'S FOOT a fungal infection usually occurring on the skin between the toes

AURA the invisible layers of subtle energy that surround a human body and are said to indicate the state of health, emotions, mind, and spirit; from the Latin word aura, meaning breeze; see also subtle energy

AUTONOMIC NERVOUS SYSTEM controls the involuntary action of internal organs, muscles, and glands

B

BILE thick, oily fluid excreted by the liver; bile helps the body digest fats

BRONCHI the main forks of the windpipe

BUNION a painful inflammation of the soft tissues around the joint between the big toe and the foot

BURSITIS inflammation of the water-filled cushions surrounding the knee (bursae)

C

CALCANEUS heel of the foot

CALLUS the hardening and thickening of the skin that occurs in parts of the body subject to constant friction

CANDIDA/CANDIDA ALBICANS fungus affecting the mucous membranes and skin; causes thrush

CARDIOVASCULAR SYSTEM the vast and intricate system of blood vessels that carries blood throughout the body

CARPAL TUNNEL SYNDROME a condition in which pressure on the median nerve, as it passes into the palm of the hand, causes pain and weakness in the fingers and thumb

CENTRAL NERVOUS SYSTEM comprising the brain and spinal cord, the central nervous system makes up one of the two main nerve systems of the body, the other being the peripheral nervous system

CEREBRAL CORTEX the thin outer layers of the brain's hemispheres

CERVICAL pertaining to the cervix, the neck of the womb

CH'I (OR QI) the Chinese term for the life force or vital energy; compare prana

CHIROPODY the diagnosis and treatment of disorders of the feet (e.g. corns and ingrowing toenails)

CHRONIC persisting for a long time, a state showing no change or very slow change

COCCYGEAL pertaining to the coccyx, a little bone at the base of the spine

COLIC abdominal pain caused by wind in the intestines

CONSTIPATION condition where evacuating the bowels is infrequent and difficult

CORN a concentrated area of hard skin that usually develops on the joints of toes

CORTISONE a naturally occurring corticosteroid used as an antiinflammatory agent

DETOXIFICATION the removal of toxins from the body

DIABETES MELLITUS condition whereby the pancreas produces little or no insulin, resulting in a high blood sugar level that could eventually lead to a hyperglecemic coma

DIAPHRAGM layer of muscles and tendons that separates the abdominal cavity from the chest cavity

DIARRHEA frequent evacuation of loose (watery) stools

DUODENUM the first stretch of the small intestine

ECZEMA term for a wide range of skin conditions

EDEMA a painless swelling caused by fluid retention beneath the skin's surface

ELEMENT the four substances believed to make up all physical matter: earth, wind, fire, and water. The Chinese believe that five elements – earth, metal, water, wood and, fire – comprise the physical world.

ENDOCRINE GLANDS the major glands of the body, which secrete hormones and release them into the body

ENDORPHINS a group of chemicals manufactured in the brain that influence the body's response to pain

ESOPHAGUS the gullet or tube that passes food to the stomach by waves of peristalsis

ESTROGEN a hormone produced by the ovary, necessary for the development of female secondary sexual characteristics

EUSTACHIAN TUBE canal from the middle ear to the back of the throat (nasopharynx)

FALLOPIAN TUBES muscular channels near the ovaries, down which the egg travels after release

FECES excrement, stools

FIBROSITIS inflammation of the body's connective tissue

FLATULENCE excessive amount of gas in stomach or intestines

G

GALL BLADDER a sac attached to the liver where bile is stored and concentrated before being released into the digestive system; bile helps to break down fats in the digestive process

GASTRITIS inflammation of the stomach lining

GASTRO-INTESTINAL relating to the stomach and intestines

GOUT inflammation in joints caused by a buildup of uric acid

H

HAMMERTOE a condition that occurs when the medial joints bend so that the toe rises above the other toes and the top joint is almost curled under

HERNIA an abnormal protrusion of the abdominal contents, usually through part of the abdominal wall

HERPES inflammation of the skin or mucous membrane with clusters of deep-seated vesicles

HOLISTIC aiming to treat the individual as an entity, incorporating body, mind, and spirit, from the Greek word holos, meaning whole

HORMONE a product of living cells that produces a specific effect on the activity cells remote from its point of origin

HYPOGLYCEMIA lowered blood sugar levels or concentration

HYPOTHALAMUS part of the brain, containing a number of centers that control functions of the body such as hunger, thirst, and temperature

I

IATROGENIC DISEASE illness that is the result of medical or surgical treatment

ILEO-CECAL VALVE controls the passage of the contents of the small intestine to the large intestine

IMMUNE SYSTEM the process within an organism whereby foreign matter is distinguished and neutralized through antibody action

J

JING a Chinese term for the vital essence that is the source of life and individual development

K

KIRLIAN PHOTOGRAPHY a process of directly recording on photographic film the electrical discharge or "aura" surrounding the human body; used as a diagnostic tool in alternative medicine

L

LACHRYMAL GLAND a gland at the outer angle of the eye that secretes tears

LIGAMENT band of tough, fibrous tissue connecting two bones at a joint (or supporting an organ of the body)

LUMBAR pertaining to the section of the spine between the lowest rib and the pelvis

LUMPECTOMY the surgical removal of a lump, caused by cancer, in the breast

LYMPH NODES small masses of specialized tissue in the lymphatic system that filter off foreign particles; often felt in the neck, armpits, groin, when enlarged through disease
LYMPHOCYTES white cells that circulate in the blood and lymph vessels and are manufactured in the bone marrow and lymph organs

MALIGNANT cancerous and possibly life-threatening
MASTOID part of the skull behind the ear that contains air spaces that communicate with the ear
ME (MYALGIC ENCEPHALITIS) a long-term postviral syndrome with chronic fatigue and muscle pain on exercise
MELANIN the dark pigment in skin, hair, etc.
MERIDIANS the channels through which vital energy flows in the body. There are 14 main meridians running to and from the hands and feet to the body or head; in Chinese acupuncture, there are 59 meridians in all; Indian medicine recognizes several hundred
METABOLISM the complex process that is the fundamental chemical expression of life itself and the means by which food is converted to energy to maintain the body
METACARPALS the bones that connect the wrist to the phalanges of the fingers
METATARSALS the bones extending the length of the foot and connecting the ankle to the toes

NEURAL/NEUROLOGICAL relating to the nervous system
NEURALGIA a stabbing pain along a nerve pathway
NORADRENALIN the chemical transmitter of the sympathetic nervous system

OSTEOPATHY a manipulative technique used on the joints and now accepted in orthodox medicine. Like chiropractic, it concentrates on the spine. Founded in the 1870s by american orthodox medical practitioner Dr. Andrew Taylor Still
OSTEOPOROSIS weakening of the bones, caused by a depletion in the level of calcium
OVARIES female reproductive glands

PANCREAS GLAND gland that secretes digestive juices; insulin, which regulates blood sugar, is made in the pancreas
PARASYMPATHETIC SYSTEM part of the autonomic nervous system, which balances or complements the sympathetic system
PARATHYROID GLANDS four small ovals of endocrine tissue that secrete the hormone that maintains the level of calcium in the blood
PATHOLOGICAL unnatural or destructive process on living tissue
PELVIS the bony cavity at the lower end of the trunk
PERICARDIUM the membrane surrounding the heart
PERIPHERAL NERVOUS SYSTEM one of the two main nerve systems of the body, whose impulses travel to and from the spine through 31 pairs of spinal nerves
PHALANGES the bones of the toes
PHLEBITIS inflammation of the veins closest to the skin
PINEAL GLAND organ in the brain that secretes melatonin (the hormone that regulates sleep patterns) into the bloodstream
PITUITARY GLAND gland at the base of the brain that regulates growth
PLANTAR WART a raised patch of white, hardened skin, usually with a dark center, that appears on the sole of the foot
POLARITY THERAPY a holistic system of healing, based upon the belief that humans are predominantly spiritual beings whose health and happiness depend upon the free flow of energy within their bodies; developed by Dr. Randolph Stone, an Austrian-born naturopath, chiropractor, and osteopath
PROGESTERONE a female sex hormone that prepares the uterus for the fertilized ovum and maintains pregnancy
PROSTATE GLAND male gland surrounding neck of bladder and urethra
PSORIASIS skin disorder causing skin to become dry or itchy

RECTUM the final part of the large intestine
REFLEX produced by or concerned with a response from a nerve center to a stimulus from without
RIGID TOE fusing of the big toe with the metatarsal bone, resulting in unnatural stiffness

SACRAL pertaining to the sacrum, a triangular bone forming the keystone of the pelvic arch
SCIATICA pain in the lower back, usually a sign of some other problem, such as a slipped disk
SEMINAL VESICLE a cavity lined with cells that secretes a fluid containing semen
SHIATSU a therapy derived from acupuncture in which pressure is applied to more than 600 acupuncture points by finger, thumb, or palm; from the Japanese word shiatsu, meaning "finger pressure"
SINUSITIS inflammation of the mucous membranes lining the sinuses (especially nasal)
SOLAR PLEXUS a radiating network of nerves behind the stomach
SPLEEN organ near the stomach in which old blood cells are broken down
STIMULUS an action, influence, or agency that arouses a response from the body
SYMPATHETIC SYSTEM part of the autonomic nervous system, which balances or complements the parasympathetic system

TALUS the ankle bone
TENDON fibrous tissue connecting muscles to other parts of the body, usually bones
TENNIS ELBOW a painful condition thought to involve inflammation of the tendons of the muscles of the forearm at the point where they join the bone of the upper arm
TESTES male reproductive organs
TESTOSTERONE the male sex hormone, which stimulates sperm production, the growth of the male genitals, and development of male "secondary characteristics"
THORACIC pertaining to the thorax or chest cavity
THROMBOSIS formation of a blood clot in a blood vessel
THYMUS GLAND gland near the root of the neck active in infancy and youth when it produces white blood cells
THYROID GLAND gland in the neck near the windpipe; it secrets the growth hormone thyroxine
TINNITUS a condition where sounds (ringing) appear in the ear for no apparent reason
TONSILS pair of small lymph nodes inside the mouth on either side of the root of the tongue; protect the throat but liable to become infected themselves
TOXIN substance that is poisonous to the body
TRACHEA windpipe
TRIPLE BURNER though there is no anatomical organ that correlates with the triple burner, the Chinese believe that all the organs in the body are guarded by it

URETER a duct that conveys urine from the kidneys to the bladder
URETHRA the canal by which urine is discharged from the bladder

VARICOSE VEINS a condition in which veins become distended and twisted, particularly in the leg
VAS DEFERENS the spermatic duct, carrying sperm from the testis to the urethra
VASCULAR pertaining to vessels conveying fluids
VISCERA the organs situated within the chest and abdomen

WEB connective tissue
WHITLOW painful inflammation of a finger or toe

YIN/YANG in the Chinese tradition, the concept of the balance between opposite principles: masculine and feminine, light and dark, positive and negative. The yin/yang symbol demonstrates how each principle contains the seed of its opposite and how both are needed to construct a rounded, balanced whole.

ZONE THERAPY the basis of modern foot reflexology, charting the feet in relation to zones of the body and their effects on the rest of the anatomy
ZONES the lines of vital energy in reflexology

BIBLIOGRAPHY

AÏVANHOV, Omraam Mikhaël, *The Zodiac, Key to Man and to the Universe*, Editions Prosveta, Fréjus, France, 1986

ARNOT, Michelle, *Foot Notes*, Sphere Books, London, 1982

BALLARD, Juliet Brooke, *The Hidden Laws of the Earth*, A.R.E. Press, Virginia Beach, Virginia, 1986

BAYLEY, Doreen, *Reflexology Today*, Thorsons, New York, 1986

BECKER, Robert, M.D. and Seldon, Gary, *The Body Electric*, Quill, William Morrow, New York, 1985

BLOFELD, John, *Taoism – The Quest for Immortality*, Unwin Paperbacks, London, 1979

BRESSLER, Harry Bond, *Zone Therapy*, Health Research, Mokelumne Hill, California, 1971

BURR, Harold Saxton, *Blueprint for Immortality*, C. W. Daniel Company, Saffron Walden, 1972

BYERS, Dwight C., *Better Health with Foot Reflexology*, Ingham Publishing, St Petersburg, Florida, 1986

CHERASKIN, E. and Ringsdorf Jr, W. M. with Brecher, Arline, *Psychodietetics*, Bantam Books, New York, 1985

CHINESE TRADITIONAL MEDICAL COLLEGE OF SHANGHAI AND CHINESE TRADITIONAL RESEARCH INSTITUTE OF SHANGHAI, *Anatomical Charts of the Acupuncture Points and 14 Meridians*, Shanghai People's Publishing House, 1976

CHOPRA, Deepak, M.D., *Perfect Health*, Bantam Books, London, 1990

CONNELLY, Dianne M., Ph.D., M.A.C., *Traditional Acupuncture: The Law of the Five Elements*, Centre for Traditional Acupuncture, Columbia, Maryland, 1989

COPEN, Bruce, Ph.D., D. Litt., *Magic of the Aura*, Academic Publications, Haywards Heath, 1976

DAVIDSON, John, *Subtle Energy*, C. W. Daniel Company, Saffron Walden, 1987

FAST, Julius, *You and Your Feet*, Pelham Books, London, 1971

FITZGERALD, William H. and Bowers, Edwin F., *Zone Therapy*, Health Research, Mokelumne Hill, California, 1917

FRYDENLUND, Jorgen, *Meridianlaren*, Forlaget Alterna

GILLANDERS, Ann, *Reflexology – The Ancient Answer to Modern Ailments*, Gillanders, 1987

GOOSMAN-LEGGER, Astrid, *Zone Therapy Using Foot Massage*, C. W. Daniel Company, Saffron Walden, 1983

GORE, Anya, *Reflexology*, Optima, London, 1990

GRINBERG, Avi, *Holistic Reflexology*, Thorsons, Wellingborough, 1989

HALL, Nicola M., *Reflexology – A Patient's Guide*, Thorsons, Wellingborough, 1986

HALL, Nicola M., *Reflexology – A Way to Better Health*, Pan Books, London, 1988

HOLFORD, Patrick, "Population Protection," *Here's Health* magazine, August 1989

INGHAM, Eunice D., *Stories the Feet Can Tell Thru Reflexology*, Ingham Publishing, St Petersburg, Florida, 1938

INGHAM, Eunice D., *Stories the Feet Have Told Thru Reflexology*, Ingham Publishing, St Petersburg, Florida, 1951

ISSEL, Christine, *Reflexology: Art, Science and History*, New Frontier Publishing, Sacramento, 1990

KAPTCHUK, Ted J., O.M.D., *The Web That Has No Weaver*, Conden & Weed, New York, 1983

KUNZ, Kevin and Barbara, *The Complete Guide to Foot Reflexology*, Thorsons, Wellingborough, 1982

LAWSON-WOOD, D. & J., *The Five Elements of Acupuncture & Chinese Massage*, Health Science Press, Devon, 1985

LEWITH, George, M.D. and Kenyon, Julian, M.D., *Clinical Ecology*, Thorsons, Wellingborough, 1985

MAARSA-TEEGURDEN, Iona, *Handbook of Acupressure II*, Ginseng du Foundation, 1981

MACDONALD, Alexander, *Acupuncture – From Ancient Art to Modern Medicine*, Unwin, London, 1982

MAJHISTTAGENMALM, *Zonterapi og Urtemeduim*, Komma Helse

MANAKA, Yoshio, M.D. and Urquhart, Ian A., Ph.D., *A Layman's Guide to Acupuncture*, Weatherhill, New York, 1972

MANN, Felix, *Acupuncture*, Pan Books, London, 1971

MARQUARDT, Hanne, *Reflex Zone Therapy of the Feet*, Thorsons, Wellingborough, 1983

MCKINLEY, Philippa, "Secrets of the Life Force", *Here's Health* magazine, January 1991

NIGHTINGALE, Michael, *Acupuncture*, Optima, London, 1987

NORMAN, Laura, *Feet First*, Simon & Schuster, New York, 1988

PIKE, Geoff, *The Power of Ch'i*, Bay Books, Sydney, 1980

RIDDLE, Janet, *Anatomy & Physiology Applied to Nursing*, Churchill Livingstone, Edinburgh, 1985

RUSSEL, Lewis and Hardy, Bob, *Healthy Feet*, Optima, London, 1988

SEEM, Mark, Ph.D. with Kaplan, Joan, *Bodymind Energetics*, Thorsons, Wellingborough, 1987

SILLS, Franklyn, *The Polarity Process*, Element Books, Shaftesbury, 1989

SOO, Chee, *The Taoist Ways of Healing*, Aquarian Press, Wellingborough, 1986

STANWAY, Dr. Andrew, *Alternative Medicine – A Guide to Natural Therapies*, Penguin Books, Harmonsdworth, 1982

THIE, John F., *Touch for Health*, T. H. Enterprises, Pasadena, California, 1973

TOFFLER, Alvin, *Future Shock*, Bodley Head, London, 1975

VEITH, Ilza, *The Yellow Emperor's Classic of Internal Medicine*, University of California Press, 1972

WAGNER, Franz, Ph.D., *Reflex Zone Massage*, Thorsons, Wellingborough, 1987

WATSON, Lyall, *Supernature*, Coronet Books, London, 1974

WATSON, Lyall, *Supernature II*, Sceptre, London, 1987

WATSON, Lyall, *Beyond Supernature*, Hodder & Stoughton, London 1986

WATSON, Lyall, *The Romeo Error*, Anchor Press/Doubleday, New York, 1974

WATSON, Lyall, *Gifts of Unknown Things*, Sceptre, London, 1987

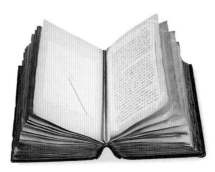

USEFUL ADDRESSES

EUROPE

DENMARK
FORENEDE DANSKE ZONETERAPEUTER
Daemningen 62, Nustrup, 6500 Vojens, Denmark
Fax 45 7487 1074

FINLAND
FINNISH ASSOCIATION OF NATURAL THERAPIES
Palvi Hannonen, Pilspan Kylantie, 01730 Vantaa, Finland

GERMANY
DEUTSCHER REFLEXOLOGEN VERBAND
Lloyd G. Wells Str., 14163 Berlin, Germany
Tel 49 30 813 10 22 Fax 49 30 813 10 27

FORTBILDUNGSZENTRUN FUR KOMPLEXE
Reflexzonentherapie, D-6232 Bad Soden, Germany

GREECE
HELLENIC ASSOCIATION OF REFLEXOLOGISTS
84 Alklonis Str., P. Faliro 17562, Athens, Greece

REPUBLIC OF IRELAND
IRISH REFLEXOLOGISTS INSTITUTE
c/o 11 Fitzwilliam Place, Dublin 2,
Republic of Ireland
Tel 353 1 760137 Fax 353 1 610466

ITALY
FEDERATZIONE ITALIANA DI REFLESSOLOGIA DEL PIEDE
Via Petrocchi 19, 20127 Milan, Italy
Tel 39 2 2822275

NETHERLANDS
VERENIGING VAN NEDERLANDS REFLEXZONE THERAPEUTEN
Noorderhaven 37A, Groningen 9712 VH, Netherlands

BOND VAN EUROPESE REFLEXOLOGEN (Society of European Reflexologists) Netherlands Section
PO Box 9009, 1006 AA Amsterdam, Netherlands
Fax 31 34 20 22178/31 20 61 76918

UK
ASSOCIATION OF REFLEXOLOGISTS
27 Old Gloucester Street, London WC1N 3XX
Tel [ring 01892 512612 at end of March for new 0990 no.]

THE BAILEY SCHOOL OF REFLEXOLOGY
Monks Orchard, Whitbourne, Worcs WR6 5RB
Tel/Fax 01886 821207

BRITISH COMPLEMENTARY MEDICINE ASSOCIATION
39 Prestbury Road, Cheltenham , Glos GL52 2PT
Tel 01242 226770 Fax 01242 226778

BRITISH SCHOOL OF REFLEXOLOGY AND HOLISTIC ASSOCIATION OF REFLEXOLOGISTS
92 Sheering Road, Old Harlow , Essex CM17 0JW
Tel 01279 429060 Fax 01279 445234

THE CHRYSALIS SCHOOL OF REFLEXOLOGY
14 Central Avenue, Cooktown, Co. Tyrone, Northern Ireland
Tel 016487 63664

COLOUR AND REFLEXOLOGY (Pauline Wills)
9 Wyndale Avenue, Kingsbury, London NW9 9PT
Tel/Fax 0181 204 7672

INTERNATIONAL FEDERATION OF REFLEXOLOGISTS
76–8 Edridge Road, Croydon, Surrey CR0 1EF
Tel 0181 667 9458 Fax 0181 649 9291

INTERNATIONAL INSTITUTE OF REFLEXOLOGY
15 Hartfield Close, Tonbridge, Kent
Tel/Fax 01732 350629

NORTH-EAST SCHOOL OF REFLEXOLOGY
30 Ridley Street, Klondyke, Cranlington, Northumberland
Tel 01670 713004

SCOTTISH INSTITUTE OF REFLEXOLOGY
(contact: Margaret Whittington)
'Taymount', Hill Crescent, Wormit, Fife BD6 8PQ
Tel 01382 541372

SCOTTISH SCHOOL OF REFLEXOLOGY
2 Wheatfield Road, Ayr KA7 2XB
Tel 01292 287142

COUNTRIES OUTSIDE EUROPE

AUSTRALIA

VICTORIAN SCHOOL OF REFLEXOLOGY AND
HERBAL STUDIES
19 Dickson Street, Sunshine , Victoria 3020, Australia
Tel 61 03 312 5573 Fax 61 03 311 3501

REFLEXOLOGY ASSOCIATION OF AUSTRALIA
15 Kedumba Crescent, Turramurra 2074,
New South Wales, Australia

CANADA

REFLEXOLOGY ASSOCIATION OF CANADA (RAC)
11 Glen Cameron Road, Unit 4, Thornhill,
Ontario L8T 4NB, Canada
Tel 1 905 889 5900

CHINA

CHINA REFLEXOLOGY ASSOCIATION
PO Box 2002, Beijing 100026, China
Fax 86 1 5068309

CHINESE SOCIETY OF REFLEXOLOGISTS
Xuanwu Hospital, Capital Institute of Medicine,
Chang Chun Street, Beijing, China

HONG KONG

RWO-SHR HEALTH INSTITUTE INTERNATIONAL
Room 1902, Java Commercial Centre,
128 Java Road, North Point, Hong Kong

ISRAEL

ISRAELI REFLEXOLOGY ASSOCIATION
PO Box 39220, Tel Aviv 61391, Israel

MALAYSIA

RWO-SHR HEALTH INSTITUTE INTERNATIONAL
1-11 Wilayah Shopping Centre, Jalan Campbell 50100,
Kuala Lumpur, Malaysia

NEW ZEALAND

THE NEW ZEALAND INSTITUTE
OF REFLEXOLOGISTS INC.
253 Mt. Albert Road, Mt. Roskill, Auckland,
New Zealand

NEW ZEALAND REFLEXOLOGY ASSOCIATION
PO Box 31 084 , Auckland 4, New Zealand

RUSSIA

I M SECHENOV MOSCOW MEDICAL ACADEMY
Dept of Complementary Medicine, B. Pirogovskaja
2/6, Moscow 119881, Russia
Tel 7 095 246 96676 Fax 7 095 248 0214

SOUTH AFRICA

THE SOUTH AFRICAN REFLEXOLOGY SOCIETY
PO Box 201858, Durban North 4016, South Africa

UNITED STATES

FOOT REFLEX AWARENESS ASSOCIATION
PO Box 7622, Mission Hills , California 91346

REFLEXOLOGY ASSOCIATION OF CALIFORNIA
PO Box 641156, Los Angeles, California 90064

ASSOCIATED REFLEXOLOGISTS
OF COLORADO
7043 West Colfax Avenue, Denver, Colorado 80215

MAINE COUNCIL OF REFLEXOLOGISTS
PO Box 969, Jefferson, Maine 04348

NEVADA REFLEXOLOGY ORGANIZATION
4186 Walhaven Court, Las Vegas, Nevada 89103
Tel 1 702 871 9522

REFLEXOLOGY ASSOCIATION OF AMERICA
4012 S. Rainbow Boulevard, Box K585,
Las Vegas, Nevada 89103-2509

REFLEXOLOGY RESEARCH PROJECT
PO Box 35820, Albuquerque, New Mexico 87176

NORTH DAKOTA REFLEXOLOGY ASSOCIATION
Route 1, Box 11, Harvey, North Dakota 58341

OHIO ASSOCIATION OF REFLEXOLOGISTS
PO Box 428725, Cincinnati, Ohio 45242

PENNSYLVANIA REFLEXOLOGY ASSOCIATION
3130 Trolley Bridge Circle, Quakertown,
Pennsylvania 18951

REFLEXOLOGY &MERIDIAN THERAPY

THE INTERNATIONAL SCHOOL OF

VACUFLEX REFLEXOLOGY SYSTEM

The International School of Reflexology & Meridian Therapy is run by author Inge Dougans, and specializes in the Vacuflex Reflexology System. It sells reflexology and meridian and five elements posters and a video entitled "The Art of Reflexology – a step-by-step guide." Its head office is in South Africa and it has branches throughout the world at the following addresses (from which a catalogue may be obtained):

HEAD OFFICE
INGE DOUGANS
PO Box 68283
Bryanston
Johannesburg 2021
South Africa
Tel/Fax 27 11 706 4206

KAREN NEL
1951 Glenarie Avenue
North Vancouver V7P 1X9
Canada
Tel 1 604 9867121

CECILE MYSLICKI
70 Parkville Drive
Winnipeg
Manitoba R2M 2H5
Canada
Tel/Fax 1 204 2539735

CAROL BOSIGER
PO Box 93
Tadworth
Surrey KT20 7YB
England
Tel/Fax 01737 842961

ANDREA SCHIPPERS
Domkeweg 23
37213 Witzenhausen
Germany
Tel 49 5542 71463

ALBERTO CARNEVALE-MAFFE
Via Procaccini 47
Milan, Italy
Tel/Fax 39 2 311116

KARINE VAN NIEKERK
Frankenstraat 31A
2582 SE Den Haag
Netherlands
Tel 31 70 3545304

LENA WALTERS
Vale Da Telha
Apartado 173
Aljezur 8670
Algarve, Portugal
Tel 351 82 98566

ANN-CHATRINE JONSSON
Värmlandsvägen 438
12348 Farsta
Sweden
Tel/Fax 46 8 942485

JILL TONKOVICH
2222 Kilkare Parkway
Pt Pleasant
New Jersey 08742
U.S.A.
Tel 1 908 8927566

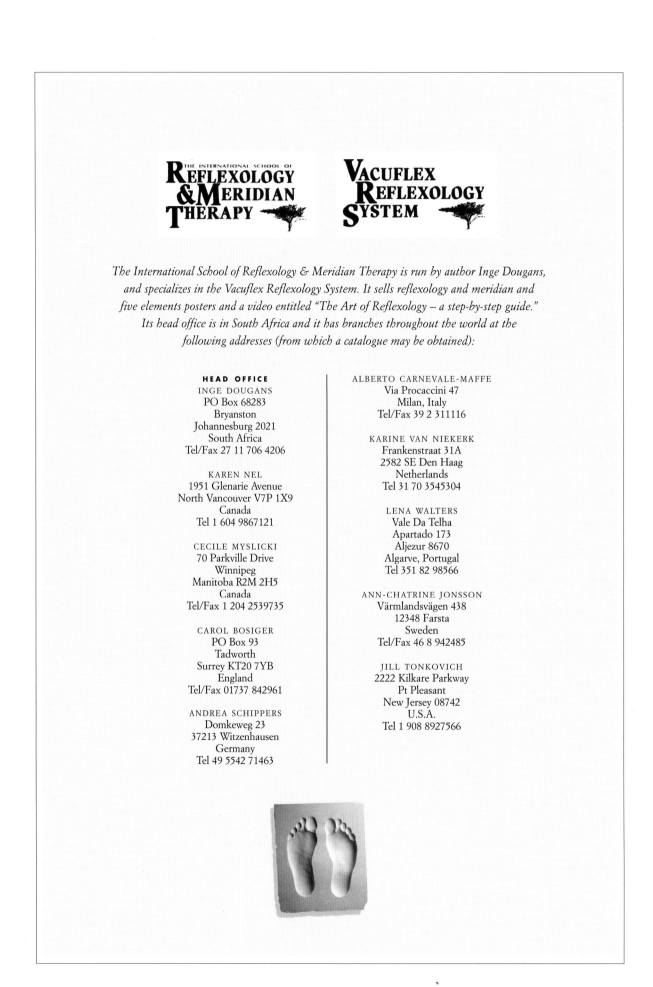

INDEX